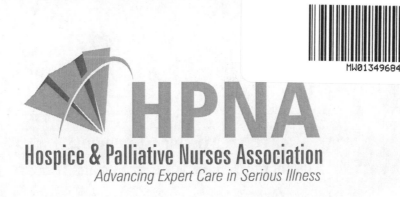

Study Guide for the Hospice and Palliative Registered Nurse

Fourth Edition

Coordinating Editors:

Patricia Berry, PhD, RN, ACHPN®, FPCN®, FAAN
Professor
Director, Hartford Center of Gerontological Nursing Excellence at OHSU
School of Nursing
Oregon Health and Science University
Portland, OR

Holli Martinez, FNP-BC, ACHPN®, FPCN®
Program Director
Palliative Care Service, University of Utah Health Care
Salt Lake City, UT

Dena Jean Sutermaster, RN, MSN, CHPN®
Education Specialist
Hospice and Palliative Nurses Association
Pittsburgh, PA

Hospice and Palliative Nurses Association
One Penn Center West, Suite 425
Pittsburgh, PA 15276-0109
www.AdvancingExpertCare.org

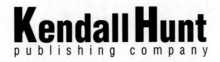

HPNA Mission Statement:

Advancing Expert Care in Serious Illness

Cover image: Mclek/Shutterstock.com

Kendall Hunt
publishing company

www.kendallhunt.com
Send all inquiries to:
4050 Westmark Drive
Dubuque, IA 52004-1840

Copyright © 2002, 2005, 2009, and 2015 by Hospice and Palliative Nurses Association

ISBN 978-1-4652-6946-1

Kendall Hunt Publishing Company has the exclusive rights to reproduce this work,
to prepare derivative works from this work, to publicly distribute this work,
to publicly perform this work and to publicly display this work.

All rights reserved. No part of this publication may be reproduced,
stored in a retrieval system, or transmitted, in any form or by any
means, electronic, mechanical, photocopying, recording, or otherwise,
without the prior written permission of the copyright owner.

Printed in the United States of America

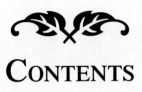

Contents

Contributors	v
Reviewers	vii
Disclaimer	ix
Introduction	xi
Part I: Study Questions and Answers	1
Part II: Case Studies for Discussion and Answers	59
Part III: Pharmacology Study Questions and Answers	87
Appendix A: Opiod Dosing Equivalence	113
Appendix B: Test Taking and Study Skills—Preparation for Success	117
Appendix C: Practice Exam	125

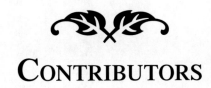

CONTRIBUTORS

Corrine Anderson, MSN, RN
Retired
Grapevine, TX

Fiona Bayne, MD
MJHS Hospice and Palliative Care
New York, NY

Patricia Berry, PhD, RN, ACHPN®, FPCN®, FAAN
Professor
Director, Hartford Center of Gerontological
　Nursing Excellence at OHSU
School of Nursing
Oregon Health and Science University
Portland, OR

Cheryl Brohard, PhD, RN, AOCN®, CHPCA®
Director of Education
Houston Hospice
Houston, TX

Margaret Donegan, MSN, APRN, NP-BC,
　ACHPN®
Nurse Practitioner, Palliative Care Team
Medical College of Wisconsin
Milwaukee, WI

Beverly J. Douglas, MSN, GNP-BC, ACHPN®,
　ARNP
Nurse Practitioner
Life Path Hospice, Division of Chapters Health
　Services
Tampa, FL

Catherine Parsons Emmett, PhD, ARNP, ACHPN®
Professional Development Facilitator, Advance
　Clinical Practice
Suncoast Hospice
Clearwater, FL

Annette M. Feierman, RN, MSN, CPHQ, CHPN®
Hospice Staff Educator
MJHS Hospice and Palliative Care
New York, NY

Colleen Fleming-Damon, PhDc, APRN,
　ACHPN®, CT
Director of Education and Training
MJHS Hospice and Palliative Care
New York, NY

Marlene A. S. Foreman, RN, BSN, ACNS-BC,
　ACHPN®
Clinical Nurse Specialist/Education Coordinator/
　Veteran Coordinator
Hospice of Acadiana, Inc.
Lafayette, LA

Nan Grottanelli, ARNP, AGPCNP-BC, CHPN®
Nurse Practitioner
Caremore
Richmond, VA

Susan Lysaght Hurley, PhD, GNP-BC, ACHPN®
Nurse Practitioner
North Shore Medical Center
Salem, MA

Sandra Jense, DNP, ACNP-BC
Nurse Practitioner
University of Utah
Salt Lake City, UT

Karen A. Kehl, PhD, RN, ACHPN®, FPCN®
Assistant Professor
University of Wisconsin-Madison, School of
　Nursing
Madison, WI

Niki Koesel, ANP, ACHPN®, FPCN®
Director of Palliative Care, Levine Cancer Institute
Carolinas Healthcare System
Charlotte, NC

Paula Larsen, LCSW, ACHP-SW
Palliative Care Social Worker
University of Utah Hospital and Clinics, Social Work Office
Salt Lake City, UT

Judith C. Lentz, RN, MSN, FPCN®
Retired
Moon Township, PA

Amy Z. McDevitt, MSN, ANP, ACHPN®
Nurse Practitioner
Roper St. Francis Healthcare
Charleston, SC

Sandra Muchka, MSN, RN, APNP, ACNS-BC, ACHPN®, FPCN®
Clinical Nurse Specialist
Froedtert Hospital
Milwaukee, WI

Judith A. Paice, PhD, RN
Director, Cancer Pain Program
Northwestern University, Feinberg School of Medicine
Chicago, IL

Deanne Sayles, RN, MN, CHPN®
Director of Quality, Education & Clinical Practice
Hinds Hospice
Fresno, CA

Pamela Shockey Stephenson, PhD, RN, AOCNS, PMHCNS-BC
Assistant Professor
Kent State University
Kent, OH

Bridget Sumser, LMSW
Director of Palliative Social Work
Winthrop University Hospital
Mineola, NY

Katherine P. Supiano, PhD, LCSW, FT, F-GSA
Associate Professor
Director, Caring Connections: A Hope & Conflict in Grief Program
University of Utah College of Nursing
Salt Lake City, UT

Sherra Stewart-Rego, RN, BSN, MPH, CHPN®
Hospice Director
VNS of Connecticut Hospice at Home
Trumbull, CT

Debbie Stoughton, RN, BSN, PHN, CHPN®
Director of Patient Care Services
Sea Crest Hospice
Costa Mesa, CA

Dena Jean Sutermaster, RN, MSN, CHPN®
Education Specialist
Hospice and Palliative Nurses Association
Pittsburgh, PA

Karen Wahle, RN, MSN, JD, CHPN®
Hospice RN
Capital Caring
Falls Church, VA

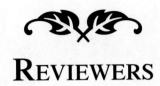

REVIEWERS

Patricia Berry, PhD, RN, ACHPN®, FPCN®, FAAN
Professor
Director, Hartford Center of Gerontological
 Nursing Excellence at OHSU
School of Nursing
Oregon Health and Science University
Portland, OR

Jennifer Fournier, APRN, MSN, ACNS-BC,
 AOCN, CHPN®
Clinical Special Services Manager
Clinical Nurse Specialist
Nancy N. and J.C. Lewis Cancer & Research
 Pavilion @ St. Joseph's/Candler
Savannah, GA

Nancy L. Grandovic, RN, BSN, MEd, CHPN®
Director of Education
Hospice and Palliative Nurses Association
Pittsburgh, PA

Nancy Joyner, APRN-CNS, ACHPN®
Palliative Care Clinical Nurse Specialist
Nancy Joyner Consulting, P.C.
Grand Forks, ND

Holli Martinez, FNP-BC, ACHPN®, FPCN®
Program Director
Palliative Care Service, University of Utah
 Health Care
Salt Lake City, UT

Barbara Schmal, MS, RN, CHPN®
Central Clinical Resource Nurse
Hospice of the Valley
Phoenix, AZ

Dena Jean Sutermaster, RN, MSN, CHPN®
Education Specialist
Hospice and Palliative Nurses Association
Pittsburgh, PA

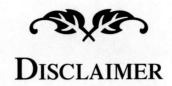

DISCLAIMER

The Hospice and Palliative Nurses Association,
its officers and directors, and the authors and reviewers of this *Study Guide*
make no claims that buying or studying this publication will guarantee a passing score
on the CHPN® Certification examination.

The Hospice and Palliative Nurses Association will not be held liable or responsible
for individual treatments, specific plans of care, or patient and family outcomes.
This *Study Guide* is intended for professional education purposes only.

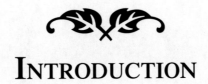

INTRODUCTION

The goal of this *Study Guide for the Hospice and Palliative Registered Nurse*, along with its companion textbook, the *Core Curriculum for the Hospice and Palliative Registered Nurse*, is to enhance existing and newly-learned principles of hospice and palliative nursing. This fourth edition of the *Study Guide* has corresponding review questions including pharmacological interventions and in-depth case studies that explore realistic clinical scenarios. See the corresponding section in the *Core Curriculum* for references.

Holli Martinez, Salt Lake City, Utah
Patricia Berry, Portland, Oregon

Study Questions
and Answers

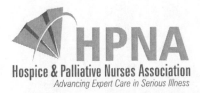

Overview of Hospice and Palliative Care

1. Where was the first palliative care program?
    A. The Connecticut Hospice, Branford, CT
    B. Hospice of the Valley, Phoenix, AZ
    C. Royal Victorian Hospital, Montreal, Canada
    D. St. Christopher's, London, England

2. An example of advocacy in hospice and palliative care is
    A. Accepting the role of an officer in your local Hospice and Palliative Nurses Association chapter.
    B. Designing a research program to compare effective pain management protocols.
    C. Explaining the latest research on a new pain management protocol to a patient.
    D. Negotiating continuous care reimbursement with a private insurance company.

3. When did hospice care become a Medicare benefit?
    A. 1971
    B. 1974
    C. 1983
    D. 1986

4. National certification is available to all roles of the hospice and palliative team **EXCEPT**
    A. Social workers.
    B. Registered nurse.
    C. Advanced practice registered nurse.
    D. Nursing assistant.

5. Aside from unspecified debility, which is the most common non-cancer hospice admitting diagnosis nationally?
    A. Lung disease
    B. Dementia
    C. Heart disease
    D. Liver disease

Study Questions and Answers • 3

1. Answer is C

    A. Incorrect: The Connecticut Hospice was the first hospice program in the United States.

    B. Incorrect: Hospice of the Valley in Phoenix, AZ, an early, very large, and well-known hospice, was founded in 1977.

    C. **Correct:** Balfour Mount, a physician, founded the first palliative care program in 1975 in Montreal and was the first to use the term "palliative."

    D. Incorrect: St. Christopher's Hospice is a hospice program located in suburban London.

2. Answer is D

    A. Incorrect: This would exemplify *leadership*.

    B. Incorrect: This leads to furthering *research* to benefit effective patient management.

    C. Incorrect: This activity is more in keeping with *education*.

    D. **Correct:** Advocacy is defined as promoting patient and family values, wishes, and preference of care, legal and ethical decision-making, and improved access to care and community resources by influencing or formulating health and social policy.

3. Answer is C

    A. Incorrect: See C.

    B. Incorrect: See C.

    C. **Correct:** In 1983, the Tax Equity Fiscal Responsibility Act created the Medicare Hospice Benefit and defined hospice care in the United States as legitimate medical care.

    D. Incorrect: See C.

4. Answer is A

    A. **Correct:** The Hospice and Palliative Credentialing Center (HPCC) formerly the National Board for Certification of Hospice and Palliative Nurses offers certification. In addition, national certification is available for the pediatric nurse, administrator, perinatal loss care provider, and the licensed practical/vocational nurse. Social workers can obtain certification as administrators and perinatal loss care providers, but not specifically for their role.

    B. Incorrect: See A.

    C. Incorrect: See A.

    D. Incorrect: See A.

5. Answer is B

    A. Incorrect: Lung disease accounts for 8.2% of hospice admitting diagnoses nationally.

    B. **Correct:** Persons with dementia comprise 15.2% of hospice diagnoses nationally with all non-cancer diagnoses at 63.5%.

    C. Incorrect: Heart disease accounts for 13.42% of hospice admitting diagnoses nationally.

    D. Incorrect: Liver disease accounts for 2.1% of hospice admitting diagnoses nationally.

6. How does hospice differ from palliative care?

   A. Hospice care is limited to the home setting.

   B. Hospice refers to care during the final stages of life; palliative care refers to care throughout the continuum of an illness.

   C. Hospice requires the patient to agree to a do not resuscitate order.

   D. Palliative care does not include the patient's family or close others.

7. To seek scholarship assistance for certification as a specialist in hospice and palliative nursing, the best source would be to apply to

   A. End-of-Life Nursing Education Consortium (ELNEC).

   B. Hospice and Palliative Credentialing Center (HPCC).

   C. Hospice and Palliative Nurses Association (HPNA).

   D. Hospice and Palliative Nurses Foundation (HPNF).

8. What is the National Consensus Project for Quality Palliative Care?

   A. A consortium of nursing organizations committed to palliative care.

   B. The basis for national certification in palliative nursing.

   C. The Joint Commission Accreditation program for palliative care programs.

   D. An organization that promotes quality palliative care, fosters consistent and high standards in palliative care, and encourages continuity of care across settings.

9. Which of the following has its roots in the early hospice movement?

   A. Care of the whole person

   B. Home-based care

   C. Reimbursement for services

   D. The use of as-needed opioid medications

6. Answer is B

    A. Incorrect: Both hospice and palliative care are delivered in any setting; only 42% of hospice patients die in their own home, defined as a private residence.

    B. **Correct:** Palliative care is not the same as end-of-life care; hospice care is palliative care as the end of life nears, usually within 6 months of death.

    C. Incorrect: While some hospices requires a do not resuscitate order for admission, not all do; such an order is not a requirement to access either hospice or palliative care.

    D. Incorrect: Both hospice and palliative care include family and close others in the approach to care.

7. Answer is D

    A. Incorrect: End-of-Life Nursing Education Consortium (ELNEC) is an education program and does not offer scholarships.

    B. Incorrect: The Hospice and Palliative Credentialing Center administers the certification exams, but does not offer scholarships.

    C. Incorrect: This membership organization has many purposes but does not offer scholarships for certification.

    D. **Correct:** The purpose of the foundation is to enhance nursing excellence with grants and scholarships for education and certification. More information can be found at www.AdvancingExpertCare.org.

8. Answer is D

    A. Incorrect: The National Consensus Project serves as a task force of the Hospice and Palliative Care Coalition comprised of 6 multidisciplinary organizations: American Academy of Hospice and Palliative Medicine (AAHPM), Center to Advance Palliative Care (CAPC), Hospice and Palliative Nurses Association (HPNA), National Association of Social Workers (NASW), National Hospice and Palliative Care Organization (NHPCO), and National Palliative Care Research Center (NPCRC).

    B. Incorrect: The basis for national certification exams is a role delineation study.

    C. Incorrect: There are separate accreditation standards for The Joint Commission Accreditation program. It is not connected to the National Consensus Project for Quality Palliative Care.

    D. **Correct:** This is the mission of the National Consensus Project for Quality Palliative Care.

9. Answer is A

    A. **Correct:** Early hospices, as early as the Middle Ages, promoted whole person care, including mind, body, soul, and spirit.

    B. Incorrect: The first formal hospice was as an inpatient program.

    C. Incorrect: The early hospice programs were religious or charity-based where care was provided free of charge for those needing it.

    D. Incorrect: Scheduled medications (or around-the-clock administration) were a feature of early hospice programs, especially those in the United Kingdom.

10. The growth in palliative care can be accounted for all of the following **EXCEPT**
    A. Acknowledgement by the healthcare system that care of those with serious illness is in need of improvement.
    B. Lessening of Centers for Medicare & Medicaid regulations.
    C. National emphasis on advance care planning.
    D. The increased interest in physician aid in dying/assisted suicide.

Interdisciplinary Collaborative Practice in the Hospice and Palliative Settings

11. Core members of the interdisciplinary team under the Medicare Hospice Benefit include
    A. Chaplain, physician, and hospice aides.
    B. Pet therapist, registered nurse, and hospice aides.
    C. Physician, nurse, medical social worker, and counseling services.
    D. Volunteers, physicians, and registered nurses.

12. Types of typical healthcare teams may include
    A. Functional and dysfunctional.
    B. Multidisciplinary, interdisciplinary, and transdisciplinary.
    C. Predisciplinary, middisciplinary, and postdisciplinary.
    D. Predisciplinary, multidisciplinary, and functional.

13. A multidisciplinary team
    A. Is comprised of several physicians within a healthcare setting.
    B. Can be organized in a hierarchical manner.
    C. Is considered to be the most effective.
    D. Operates solely in a hospital setting.

10. Answer is B
    A. Incorrect: This is a reason for the growth in palliative care.
    B. **Correct:** Centers for Medicare & Medicaid do not regulate palliative care.
    C. Incorrect: This is a reason for the growth in palliative care.
    D. Incorrect: This is a reason for the growth in palliative care.

Interdisciplinary Collaborative Practice in the Hospice and Palliative Settings

11. Answer is C
    A. Incorrect: See C.
    B. Incorrect: See C.
    C. **Correct:** A physician, nurse, medical social worker, and counseling services are the core members of the Hospice Medicare Benefit interdisciplinary team. Other team members can be added as needed.
    D. Incorrect: See C.

12. Answer is B
    A. Incorrect: These are not types of healthcare teams.
    B. **Correct:** The 3 common types of healthcare teams are multidisciplinary, interdisciplinary, and transdisciplinary.
    C. Incorrect: These are not types of healthcare teams.
    D. Incorrect: Of this list, only multidisciplinary is a type of healthcare team.

13. Answer is B
    A. Incorrect: Team members are from multiple disciplines.
    B. **Correct:** Multidisciplinary team members can be organized in hierarchical manner.
    C. Incorrect: This is not true as the hierarchical manner can result in limited sharing of decisions and leadership as well as having limited coordination and consultation between the disciplines.
    D. Incorrect: Multidisciplinary teams are not limited to any one setting.

14. According to the Medicare Hospice Benefit, how often must the interdisciplinary group review, revise, and document the individualized plan?

    A. As often as all members of the team can meet together in one room.

    B. At least every 15 days.

    C. Only with changes in the patient's condition.

    D. There are no regulations on how often the team must meet.

15. Which of the following best reflects the definition of a peer review?

    A. A passive method of supporting clinicians with less experience.

    B. A process by which clinicians are held accountable for their practice.

    C. Direct supervision of a clinician.

    D. Long-term relationship between experienced and less-experienced clinicians.

16. Volunteers

    A. Are required by the Hospice Medicare Benefit.

    B. Do not need orientation and training.

    C. Provide care including bathing and toileting.

    D. Are not members of the interdisciplinary team.

17. Compassion fatigue differs from posttraumatic stress disorder in that compassion fatigue

    A. Applies to those emotionally affected by the trauma of another.

    B. Is beyond the common stressors of palliative care.

    C. Results from experiencing a trauma.

    D. Results from cynicism and depersonalization in the workplace.

14. Answer is B

    A. Incorrect: There is no provision that team meetings must be face-to-face.

    B. **Correct:** According to the Hospice Medicare Benefit, the hospice interdisciplinary group (in collaboration with the individual's attending physician, if any) must review, revise, and document the individualized plan as frequently as the patient requires, but no less frequently than every 15 calendar days.

    C. Incorrect: See B.

    D. Incorrect: In a palliative care setting, there is no stipulation on how often the team must meet, but there is in hospice care. See B.

15. Answer is B

    A. Incorrect: This describes a role model.

    B. **Correct:** This is the definition of peer review—a collegial, systematic, and periodic process by which clinicians are held accountable for practice and that fosters the refinement of one's knowledge, skills, and decision-making at all levels and in all areas of practice.

    C. Incorrect: This describes precepting.

    D. Incorrect: This describes a mentor.

16. Answer is A

    A. **Correct:** The Centers for Medicare & Medicaid Services do require volunteers to be part of the hospice interdisciplinary team.

    B. Incorrect: Hospice volunteer must receive "orientation and training that is consistent with hospice industry standards."

    C. Incorrect: Bathing and toileting are care that is provided by the nursing assistant. Volunteers can provide companionship, make deliveries, run errands, etc.

    D. Incorrect: See A.

17. Answer is A.

    A. **Correct:** Compassion fatigue is almost identical to posttraumatic stress disorder (PTSD), except that it applies to those emotionally affected by the trauma of another (usually a patient or family member).

    B. Incorrect: Compassion fatigue stems from common stressors in palliative care.

    C. Incorrect: PTSD results from an exposure to a serious threat of death, injury, or sexual trauma.

    D. Incorrect: Compassion fatigue extends beyond negative attitudes.

18. When team members do not agree on the plan of care, which of the following would be a first step for the leader to take in resolving the disagreement?

    A. Listening to all team members' concerns.

    B. Consult with the ethics committee.

    C. The senior members of the team will choose the correct plan of care.

    D. Resolve the disagreements outside of the team meetings.

Patterns of Disease Progression

19. A 56-year-old woman is referred to hospice for a diagnosis of stage IV breast cancer with metastatic disease to the lung. She reports anxiety about ongoing spread of her disease and wants to know what symptoms to be aware of that may indicate further disease progression. Based on the patterns of common disease spread, what symptoms would be most worrisome?

    A. Bone pain, superficial skin lesions, malignant bowel obstruction.

    B. Bone pain, visual disturbances, shortness of breath.

    C. Shortness of breath, malignant bowel obstruction, decreased urinary output (renal failure).

    D. Superficial skin lesions, shortness of breath, cardiac instability.

20. Chemotherapy given to a patient with colon cancer prior to surgical resection is known as what type of therapy?

    A. Adjuvant

    B. Curative

    C. Neoadjuvant

    D. Palliative

21. Which factor is the most significant in prognostication in patients with a cancer diagnosis?

    A. Brain metastases

    B. Family history of stage IV cancer

    C. Functional status

    D. Partial response to chemotherapy

18. Answer is A
    A. **Correct:** It is important that all team members' concerns be heard.
    B. Incorrect: An ethics committee consult may be needed, but it is not the first step.
    C. Incorrect: No one team member's opinion is valued above another's.
    D. Incorrect: Team meetings should be used to address all issues and conflicts.

Patterns of Disease Progression

19. Answer is B
    A. Incorrect: Skin and bowel are not common sites of metastatic spread in breast cancer.
    B. **Correct:** Three of the four most common sites of metastatic disease in breast cancer are bone, brain, and lung.
    C. Incorrect: Renal and bowel are not common sites of metastatic spread in breast cancer.
    D. Incorrect: Skin and cardiac are not common sites of metastatic spread in breast cancer.

20. Answer is C
    A. Incorrect: Adjuvant therapy is given concurrent with the primary mode of treatment.
    B. Incorrect: Curative treatment can include 2 modalities of treatment though the definition of neoadjuvant is more correct.
    C. **Correct:** Neoadjuvant therapy is defined as treatment given prior to the primary treatment.
    D. Incorrect: These modalities could be palliative in nature but the definition of neoadjuvant is more correct in this question.

21. Answer is C
    A. Incorrect: Brain metastasis alone is not the most significant factor in prognostication.
    B. Incorrect: Family history does influence risk of cancer but does not serve as a prognostic tool.
    C. **Correct:** Literature shows the patient's functional status is the most significant predictor in treatment tolerance and in overall survival.
    D. Incorrect: Partial response to treatment is not the most significant factor.

22. A registered nurse is caring for a 67-year-old man with non-small cell lung cancer in the home. Upon assessment, the nurse is concerned about possible spinal cord compression due to several new symptom reports. Which symptom is most commonly reported first in the case of spinal cord compression?

    A.   Back pain

    B.   Neurogenic bladder

    C.   Numbness of the lower extremities

    D.   Paralysis

23. The assessment of a patient reveals that the patient's right-sided heart failure symptoms are increasing. Symptoms of right-sided heart failure include

    A.   Dependent edema, nausea, and ascites.

    B.   Dyspnea, restlessness, and tachycardia.

    C.   Orthopnea, weakness, and anxiety.

    D.   Weight gain, fatigue, and cough.

24. Jack has been seen by the outpatient palliative care nurse for a serious subarachnoid aneurysm. The nurse receives a call that he is in the emergency room comatose but with stable vital signs. The most immediate response to a hemorrhagic stroke (i.e., aneurysm) is

    A.   Preserve as much brain function as possible.

    B.   Prevent complications of immobility.

    C.   Reassure the family that the patient will recover.

    D.   Rehabilitate to improve residual function.

25. Hospice eligibility guidelines for persons with neurodegenerative diseases include

    A.   Immobility, dyspnea, and aspiration.

    B.   Infections, incontinence, and barrel chest.

    C.   Secretions, decreased verbalizations, and edema.

    D.   Weight loss, decreased albumin, and rapid functional decline.

22. Answer is A

    A. **Correct:** Back pain is the most common presentation of spinal cord compression (SCC).

    B. Incorrect: Neurogenic bladder is not always associated with SCC and, if so, it will not be the first symptom.

    C. Incorrect: Numbness of extremities is typically a later symptom of SCC.

    D. Incorrect: Paralysis is a late and sometime irreversible factor in SCC.

23. Answer is A

    A. **Correct:** As systemic congestion occurs in right-sided heart failure, symptoms include weight gain, dependent peripheral edema, ascites, weakness, anorexia, and nausea.

    B. Incorrect: Dyspnea, restlessness, and tachycardia are symptoms of left-sided heart failure.

    C. Incorrect: Left-sided heart failure causes lung congestion, which leads to orthopnea, dyspnea, and anxiety.

    D. Incorrect: Fatigue and cough are symptoms of left-sided heart failure, although some patients have both at end of life.

24. Answer is A

    A. **Correct:** In the emergency room, it is imperative to initiate medications and treatments to preserve as much brain function as possible.

    B. Incorrect: Immobility may result from residual functional deficits, and correct positioning and prevention of pressure ulcers should start as soon as possible following the crisis.

    C. Incorrect: In a hemorrhagic stroke or aneurysm, it is difficult to predict if the bleeding will continue or recur, so it is too soon to reassure the family of recovery.

    D. Incorrect: Rehabilitation will occur after the immediate emergency is over and the patient is stabilized.

25. Answer is D

    A. Incorrect: Many persons with amyotrophic lateral sclerosis (ALS) and dementia may be immobile and bedbound long before they become hospice eligible.

    B. Incorrect: Barrel chest occurs in emphysema.

    C. Incorrect: Although increased secretions may occur as patients are dying, edema is not criteria for hospice admission in neurodegenerative disease.

    D. **Correct:** It is difficult to determine when a neurodegenerative disease becomes terminal, but there are hospice indicators such as rapid progression of symptoms, breathing difficulties, infections, diminished nutrition with weight loss and decreased albumin, sepsis. Use of scales such as Karnofsky, Palliative Performance Scale, and FAST are helpful.

26. The major medication groups used to manage dyspnea in chronic lung conditions at the end of life include

   A. Antibiotics and steroids.

   B. Bronchodilators and atropine.

   C. Opioids and anxiolytics.

   D. Oxygen and antidepressants.

27. Which of the following symptoms must be closely monitored and managed in palliative care for all neurodegenerative diseases?

   A. Constipation

   B. Dementia

   C. Dyspnea

   D. Immobility

28. Which of the following is a terminal event of end stage liver disease?

   A. Ascites

   B. Bleeding

   C. Hepatitis

   D. Jaundice

29. Late-stage human immunodeficiency virus (HIV) is diagnosed when the CD4 count is less than

   A. 100 cells/mm^3.

   B. 200 cells/mm^3.

   C. 300 cells/mm^3.

   D. 500 cells/mm^3.

26. Answer is C

    A. Incorrect: Steroids may help manage chronic pulmonary conditions and antibiotics are used for infections, but are not drugs of choice for dyspnea from any cause.

    B. Incorrect: Atropine is used to reduce secretions. It has little effect on dyspnea, shortness of breath.

    C. **Correct:** The most effective medication groups for relief of dyspnea are opioids and anxiolytics (usually morphine and lorazepam).

    D. Incorrect: Oxygen may be used but is not a medication group. Anxiolytics may be necessary but not all persons need antidepressants, and this would not treat dyspnea.

27. Answer is A

    A. **Correct:** Constipation is common in all neurodegenerative diseases because of decreased mobility, cognitive impairment, drooling in Parkinson's disease, and weakened muscle tone.

    B. Incorrect: Dementia is not common in amyotrophic lateral sclerosis (ALS) or multiple sclerosis (MS), although may occur with Parkinson's disease.

    C. Incorrect: Dyspnea is common in some neurodegenerative diseases such as ALS or MS, but not usually dementia.

    D. Incorrect: Some persons with dementia are mobile until near death.

28. Answer is B

    A. Incorrect: Ascites usually occurs in hepatic cirrhosis quite early in the disease. It can be managed by paracentesis or medications.

    B. **Correct:** One possible terminal event in liver disease is bleeding from gastrointestinal or esophageal varices.

    C. Incorrect: Hepatitis (especially B and C) is a cause of end stage liver disease, but persons may live a long time with hepatitis.

    D. Incorrect: Jaundice may occur even in acute hepatitis where recovery is expected.

29. Answer is B

    A. Incorrect: See B.

    B. **Correct:** Late-stage human immunodeficiency virus (HIV) or AIDS is diagnosed when CD4 count is less than 200 cells/mm^3.

    C. Incorrect: See B.

    D. Incorrect: See B.

30. Which of the following is one of the hospice eligibility criteria for human immunodeficiency virus (HIV)?

    A. Artificial nutrition is needed to maintain weight.

    B. CD4 count less than 200 cells/mm^3.

    C. Discontinuing cytomegalovirus medications.

    D. Viral load greater than 100,000 copies/mL.

Pain

31. Signs and symptoms of opioid abstinence include

    A. Anxiety, nausea, and lacrimation.

    B. Bradycardia, myoclonus, and euphoria.

    C. Hypotension, abdominal cramping, and insomnia.

    D. Sedation, diarrhea, and rhinorrhea.

32. Pain that is poorly localized, cramping, and referred to distant sites is usually

    A. Breakthrough.

    B. Neuropathic.

    C. Nociceptive.

    D. Visceral.

33. Which statement is most accurate regarding acetaminophen?

    A. Is analgesic, antipyretic, and anti-inflammatory.

    B. Is hepatotoxic in high doses and can compromise renal function.

    C. The maximum dose in combination opioid products is 500 mg.

    D. The maximum dose in 24 hours is 4000 mg/day.

30. Answer is D

    A. Incorrect: Weight loss will occur usually early in the disease and may not be able to be reversed even with artificial nutrition.

    B. Incorrect: The hospice criterion is CD4 count less than 25 cells/mm^3.

    C. Incorrect: Although other antiretrovirals may be discontinued when a person enters hospice, medications to prevent or manage cytomegalovirus retinitis is usually continued.

    D. **Correct:** One of the criteria for hospice eligibility is a viral load of greater than 100,000 copies/mL.

Pain

31. Answer is A

    A. **Correct:** These are signs and symptoms of opioid withdrawal.

    B. Incorrect: Myoclonus can be a sign of opioid abstinence but tachycardia and dysphoria are also common.

    C. Incorrect: Abdominal cramping and insomnia are correct; hypertension is more common.

    D. Incorrect: Although diarrhea and rhinorrhea are signs of opioid abstinence, sedation is not. Agitation is more common.

32. Answer is D

    A. Incorrect: Breakthrough pain is incidental, idiopathic, or can occur as end-of-dose failure.

    B. Incorrect: Neuropathic pain is usually described as tingling, burning, electrical, or shooting.

    C. Incorrect: Nociceptive pain is generally well localized and described as aching or throbbing.

    D. **Correct:** These are characteristics of visceral pain.

33. Answer is B

    A. Incorrect: Acetaminophen is not anti-inflammatory.

    B. **Correct:** These are potential toxicities of acetaminophen.

    C. Incorrect: The maximum dose of acetaminophen in prescription-based combination opioid products is now 325 mg.

    D. Incorrect: Most sources now recommend a maximum dose of 3000 mg/day of acetaminophen for chronic use.

34. Nonsteroidal anti-inflammatory drugs can
    A. Cause gastrointestinal bleeding that can be prevented with H_2 blockers.
    B. Decrease platelet numbers.
    C. Increase cardiovascular events, including myocardial infarction and stroke, in those at risk.
    D. Produce pain relief without a ceiling dose.

35. Opioid-induced respiratory depression
    A. Can be effectively monitored with intermittent pulse oximetry.
    B. Occurs more often in those with obstructive sleep apnea.
    C. Occurs when CO_2 receptors cannot sense decreasing CO_2 levels.
    D. Should be treated with rapid bolus of naloxone in opioid dependent patients.

36. Opioids can be given by a variety of routes of administration. Which of these statements is true?
    A. Subcutaneous morphine has a delayed peak effect when compared with intravenous injections.
    B. Sublingual and buccal morphine are absorbed primarily via the oral mucosa.
    C. Rectal placement of long-acting morphine produces similar levels to the oral route of administration.
    D. Transdermal fentanyl should not be used in cachectic patients.

37. Antiepileptic drugs are effective for neuropathic pain. Which statement is true regarding these agents?
    A. Carbamazepine can cause hepatotoxicity.
    B. Phenytoin causes bone marrow suppression.
    C. Pregabalin has better bioavailability than gabapentin and can be given twice a day.
    D. Monitoring of drug levels is required for all of the above antiepileptic drugs.

34. Answer is C
    A. Incorrect: Nonsteroidal anti-inflammatory drugs (NSAIDs) can increase risk of gastrointestinal bleeding but this cannot be prevented with an H_2 blocker; proton pump inhibitors or misoprostol can prevent gastrointestinal bleeding from NSAIDs.
    B. Incorrect: NSAIDs decrease the ability of platelets to clot but do not alter the numbers of platelets.
    C. **Correct:** NSAIDs can increase the risk of myocardial infarction (MI) and stroke in people at risk for cardiovascular events.
    D. Incorrect: NSAIDs do have a ceiling dose, where increases do not provide additional analgesia.

35. Answer is B
    A. Incorrect: Intermittent pulse oximetry can cause the patient to be aroused with a deep breath, providing a falsely increased oxygen reading.
    B. **Correct:** Obstructive sleep apnea (OSA) is a risk factor for opioid-induced respiratory depression.
    C. Incorrect: Carbon dioxide receptors cannot sense *increasing* CO_2 levels.
    D. Incorrect: Naloxone should be slowly titrated to treat respiratory depression without producing abstinence syndrome.

36. Answer is A
    A. **Correct:** A subcutaneous bolus of morphine peaks in approximately 30 minutes, whereas an intravenous bolus of morphine peaks in approximately 15 minutes.
    B. Incorrect: Sublingual and buccal morphine is absorbed primarily via the gastrointestinal tract.
    C. Incorrect: Rectal delivery of long acting morphine produces lower serum levels when compared with oral delivery.
    D. Incorrect: Transdermal fentanyl is less efficiently absorbed in cachectic patients when compared with the normally weighted, but meaningful levels of fentanyl can still be obtained.

37. Answer is C
    A. Incorrect: Carbamazepine can cause bone marrow suppression.
    B. Incorrect: Phenytoin can cause hepatotoxicity.
    C. **Correct:** Pregabalin can be administered 2 or 3 times a day, whereas gabapentin should be administered 3 times per day.
    D. Incorrect: Drug level monitoring is not necessary for gabapentin or pregabalin.

38. Antidepressants are useful in relieving neuropathic pain. Which statement is true?

    A. Amitriptyline has significant anticholinergic effects and is not considered first line therapy as a result.

    B. Analgesia is often seen immediately after the first dose of nortriptyline.

    C. Serotonin-norepinephrine reuptake inhibitors have little role in treating neuropathy but can be useful in the management of depression or hot flashes.

    D. Serotonin selective reuptake inhibitors such as paroxetine are effective in treating neuropathic pain.

39. Corticosteroids, such as dexamethasone

    A. Can be sedating.

    B. Can provide prolonged, improved appetite.

    C. Can relieve bone pain and right upper quadrant pain associated with liver metastases.

    D. Should be given twice a day to ensure adequate drug levels.

40. Principles of opioid use include

    A. More than 3 rescue doses per day leads to increase in the long-acting opioid dose.

    B. Reducing the dose by approximately 25% after performing an equianalgesic conversion accounts for incomplete cross-tolerance.

    C. The peak effect of immediate release oral morphine is approximately 1 hour; doses should be ordered every 3 hours to ensure drug has been metabolized.

    D. Using 50% to 100% of the daily oral opioid route produces the appropriate oral breakthrough dose.

Symptom Management

41. What is the hallmark sign of delirium?

    A. Alteration in consciousness

    B. Feeling of hopelessness

    C. Loss of memory

    D. Unable to understand something clearly

38. Answer is A

    A. **Correct:** Amitriptyline is not recommended as first line therapy.

    B. Incorrect: Analgesia is seen after 3 to 7 days.

    C. Incorrect: Serotonin-norepinephrine reuptake inhibitor (SNRI) drugs are useful in treating neuropathy, depression, and hot flashes.

    D. Incorrect: Serotonin selective reuptake inhibitor (SSRI) agents have little analgesic effect despite being effective antidepressants.

39. Answer is C

    A. Incorrect: Dexamethasone is generally activating; this increased sense of energy is a beneficial side effect.

    B. Incorrect: Dexamethasone can improve appetite but this effect is generally short lived.

    C. **Correct:** Dexamethasone is useful in treating these painful conditions.

    D. Incorrect: Dexamethasone has a long half-life and can be given once daily when used for pain control; this precludes activation that impairs sleep.

40. Answer is B

    A. Incorrect: More than 3 rescue doses per day should initiate assessment and may warrant an increase in the long-acting opioid, but this should not be automatic. An example where this should not be done is when the patient is generally comfortable most of the day but has painful dressing changes—increasing the baseline dose may result in sedation.

    B. **Correct:** A 25% reduction accounts for incomplete cross-tolerance.

    C. Incorrect: While the peak effect of immediate release oral morphine is approximately 1 hour, dosing can safely be done every 1 to 2 hours.

    D. Incorrect: The oral breakthrough dose is usually 10% to 20% of the 24-hour oral opioid dose.

Symptom Management

41. Answer is A

    A. **Correct:** An acute change in level of arousal is the hallmark indicator of delirium.

    B. Incorrect: Hopelessness is more characteristic of depression.

    C. Incorrect: Memory loss is more characteristic of dementia.

    D. Incorrect: Inability to understand something clearly is a vague description that could be seen in delirium, but is not the hallmark indicator.

42. A patient is reporting that myoclonus is causing him distress. What nonpharmacological intervention should be added to the management plan?

    A. Initiate a fan to improve airflow in the room.

    B. Request a physical therapy consult for strengthening.

    C. Try to immobilize the affected area.

    D. Use gentle massage to the affected area.

43. A patient needs education regarding healthy sleep practices. Which of the following is an appropriate intervention to include in her teaching?

    A. Change the time you go to bed every night.

    B. Eat a heavy meal 2 hours before bedtime.

    C. Exercise in the evening 2 hours before bedtime.

    D. Listen to calming music or meditate prior to bedtime.

44. What is the most important piece of information when assessing dyspnea?

    A. Lung sounds

    B. Oxygen saturation

    C. Patient's level of distress

    D. What medications are they taking

45. Family members are concerned that giving morphine to relieve dyspnea will accelerate the dying process. Which response is most appropriate?

    A. "Given in appropriate doses, morphine will slow respirations and relieve the feeling of air hunger."

    B. "Morphine is given to slow breathing but if the patient stops breathing following a dose, it is likely because they were in the process of dying."

    C. "The dose given for dyspnea is much less than the dose they are taking already for pain, so that should not be a concern."

    D. "Other opioids, such as oxycodone, could be used."

42. Answer is D

    A. Incorrect: Using a room fan will not help treat/relieve myoclonus.
    B. Incorrect: If the myoclonus is distressing, attempting physical therapy for exercise and strengthening could cause more discomfort. Once the myoclonus is under control, a physical therapy consult may be appropriate for strengthening.
    C. Incorrect: Immobilizing the area could cause more discomfort. Instead, try to reposition the patient for comfort.
    D. **Correct:** Gentle massage may help with muscle relaxation and is an appropriate intervention.

43. Answer is D

    A. Incorrect: The best routine is to get up and go to bed at the same time every day.
    B. Incorrect: The best routine is to not eat heavily for 3 hours before bedtime. A light bedtime snack is appropriate.
    C. Incorrect: It is best to limit exercise 4 hours before bedtime. It is best to engage in light exercise or increase activity in the morning or afternoon.
    D. **Correct:** Listening to calming music, meditation, reading something soothing, or taking a hot bath are all examples of ways to help relax prior to bedtime.

44. Answer is C

    A. Incorrect: Lung auscultation may identify a reversible cause but may not directly correlate to symptom distress.
    B. Incorrect: Oxygen saturation may identify a reversible cause but may not directly correlate with symptom distress.
    C. **Correct:** Dyspnea is a subjective symptom reported by the patient.
    D. Incorrect: Medication management errors may identify a reversible cause but do not directly correlate to symptom distress.

45. Answer is A

    A. **Correct:** Morphine's response is dose dependent and families should be reassured that starting with low doses and taking as prescribed would not hasten death.
    B. Incorrect: Although there may be a last dose of morphine given prior to death, this statement does not reflect the nurse's role of teaching as to the safety of morphine.
    C. Incorrect: There is no need to give less than the dose currently being used to manage pain.
    D. Incorrect: All opioids have the same side effect profile. Switching from morphine to oxycodone does not diminish the risk for respiratory depression, which is primarily dose related.

46. What stage is a pressure ulcer with skin that is red and blistered?

    A. Stage I

    B. Stage II

    C. Stage III

    D. Stage IV

47. Which of the following is an irreversible cause of anorexia-cachexia?

    A. Metastatic pancreatic cancer

    B. Refractory pain

    C. Severe depression

    D. Systemic chemotherapy

48. Which of the following is a nonpharmacological treatment for nausea and vomiting?

    A. Avoid being too relaxed before meals.

    B. Encourage large meals.

    C. Season meals with salt.

    D. Serve meals at room temperature.

49. Which of the following treatments is required for opioid-induced constipation?

    A. Bisacodyl suppository after 3 days without a bowel movement.

    B. Increase fluid and fiber intake.

    C. Increase mobility and activity.

    D. Stool softener and stimulant laxative daily.

50. What is the cause of hiccoughs in a patient who has ascites?

    A. Gastric distention

    B. Inflammation

    C. Phrenic and vagus nerve irritation

    D. Metabolic syndrome

46. Answer is B

    A. Incorrect: Stage I pressure ulcer is nonblanchable erythema. Redness surrounding blisters may be stage I, but wounds are classified by the deepest level of injury.

    B. **Correct:** Stage II pressure ulcers are partial loss of dermis as in the case of a blister.

    C. Incorrect: Stage III pressure ulcers are full thickness loss of skin.

    D. Incorrect: Stage IV pressure ulcers are full thickness tissue loss.

47. Answer is A

    A. **Correct:** Metastatic pancreatic cancer is in its most advanced stage and is not curable or reversible. In addition, pancreatic cancer can have direct effects on digestion and advanced cancer can cause metabolic abnormalities leading to anorexia-cachexia.

    B. Incorrect: If a patient is experiencing high levels of pain, it may cause decreasing appetite, therefore leading to anorexia. Pain should be assessed and treated accordingly. Once pain is improved, appetite should improve.

    C. Incorrect: If a patient is depressed, appetite may be decreased leading to anorexia. Depression should be assessed and treated accordingly. Once resolved, appetite can improve.

    D. Incorrect: Chemotherapy may temporarily cause anorexia but typically resolves once treatment is complete.

48. Answer is D

    A. Incorrect: Relaxation and guided imagery has shown to decrease nausea and vomiting.

    B. Incorrect: Small meals, slow eating, and sitting upright are all measures that can help decrease nausea and vomiting during mealtime.

    C. Incorrect: Fatty, spicy, and salty foods can cause increased nausea and vomiting.

    D. **Correct:** Food at room temperature can help decrease nausea during mealtime.

49. Answer is D

    A. Incorrect: Opioid-induced constipation needs to be treated prophylactically.

    B. Incorrect: Increasing fluids and foods high in fiber can help reduce and prevent constipation, though more is needed for opioid-induced constipation.

    C. Incorrect: Increasing mobility and activity can help reduce and prevent constipation, but will not alleviate opioid-induced constipation alone.

    D. **Correct:** A stool softener and stimulant laxative are needed to stimulate a bowel movement.

50. Answer is C

    A. Incorrect: Gastric distention is also caused by irritation of the phrenic and vagus nerves.

    B. Incorrect: Inflammation is not a cause of hiccoughs with ascites.

    C. **Correct:** Ascites can cause hiccoughs by irritating the phrenic and vagus nerves.

    D. Incorrect: Metabolic syndrome is not related to ascites.

51. Which statement best describes what to teach a patient on how to treat dry itchy skin?

   A.   "Apply alcohol-based lotions several times a day."

   B.   "Apply moisturizer over damp skin after bathing."

   C.   "Avoid menthol medicated moisturizers."

   D.   "Take a hot shower."

Psychiatric/Psychological Symptoms and Diagnoses

52. A patient treated for a known psychosis exhibits uncontrollable muscle movements and spasms around the mouth. The patient is most likely experiencing

   A.   A grand mal seizure.

   B.   Heroin withdrawal.

   C.   Hyperexcitability.

   D.   Tardive dyskinesia.

53. Signs of posttraumatic stress disorder include

   A.   Anxiety, amnesia, and dreamlessness.

   B.   Anxiety, intrusive memories, and distressing dreams.

   C.   Depression, avoidance, and lethargy.

   D.   Depression, flashbacks, and hypoexcitability.

54. A delusion in which the individual is preoccupied with their state of health is a

   A.   Control delusion.

   B.   Erotomanic delusion.

   C.   Nihilistic delusion.

   D.   Somatic delusion.

55. A patient tells the nurse "I need the voices in my head to stop yelling so loud." Based on this statement, the first thing the nurse should do is

   A.   Ask the patient if she can talk to the voices.

   B.   Ask the patient what the voices are saying.

   C.   Get an order to increase the patient's anxiolytics.

   D.   Restrict visitors until the voices subside.

51. Answer is B

    A.   Incorrect: Alcohol-based lotions can cause pruritus.

    B.   **Correct:** Applying moisturizer over damp skin helps keep the skin moister.

    C.   Incorrect: Menthol medicated moisturizers may decrease pruritus.

    D.   Incorrect: Showers and bath water temperatures should be tepid.

Psychiatric/Psychological Symptoms and Diagnoses

52. Answer is D

    A.   Incorrect: Grand mal seizures include generalized muscle spasms.

    B.   Incorrect: Heroin withdrawal is not typically associated with muscle spasms of the mouth.

    C.   Incorrect: Hyperexcitability includes heightened levels of activity and restlessness but is not typically associated with muscle spasms.

    D.   **Correct:** Uncontrollable muscle movements and spasms around the mouth are classic signs of tardive dyskinesia. It is also associated with antipsychotic medications.

53. Answer is B

    A.   Incorrect: Amnesia and dreamlessness are not hallmark signs of posttraumatic stress disorder.

    B.   **Correct:** Anxiety, intrusive memories, and distressing dreams are all hallmark signs of posttraumatic stress disorder.

    C.   Incorrect: Lethargy is not a hallmark sign of posttraumatic stress disorder.

    D.   Incorrect: Hypoexcitability is not a hallmark sign of posttraumatic stress disorder.

54. Answer is D

    A.   Incorrect: Delusions of control are the belief that an outside force is controlling the individual.

    B.   Incorrect: Erotomanic delusions are the false belief that another person is in love with the individual.

    C.   Incorrect: Nihilistic delusions are the conviction that a major catastrophe will occur.

    D.   **Correct:** Preoccupation with health is a sign of somatic delusions.

55. Answer is B

    A.   Incorrect: Communication strategies should not include accepting the voice as being real.

    B.   **Correct:** Asking the patient what the voices are saying is important to assess the risk of violence or self-harm from command hallucinations.

    C.   Incorrect: Anxiolytics are not an effective treatment for psychosis and should not be the first nursing intervention.

    D.   Incorrect: Restricting visitors is not an effective strategy for managing psychosis.

56. The nurse arrives at the home of a new hospice patient but has difficulty walking through the house because of the amount of clutter stacked in the family room and kitchen. The most likely reason for this is that the patient is

    A. Actively sorting through belongings to give to loved ones.

    B. Debilitated and unable to care for self.

    C. Exhibiting a type of obsessive-compulsive disorder.

    D. Having difficulty separating with belongings while dying.

57. A patient living in a group home with a known history of borderline personality disorder and end stage lung cancer is admitted to an inpatient hospice unit with complaints of poor pain control. The nurse understands that

    A. Patients with a psychiatric history often have undertreated pain.

    B. Patients with borderline personality disorder have lower than normal pain thresholds.

    C. The patient is probably drug seeking.

    D. The patient should be given haloperidol for breakthrough pain.

58. A male patient was admitted to the hospice service with stage IV liver cancer. His sister is staying with him to provide care. She contacts the registered nurse on call reporting that her brother did not sleep the night before as he was shaky, sweaty, agitated, and swatting at imaginary bugs in his bed. The nurse should first

    A. Assess the patient for resistant neuropathic pain.

    B. Assess the patient's history of alcohol use.

    C. Instruct the sister to administer acetaminophen for fever.

    D. Instruct the sister to dial 911.

59. The nurse visits a 72-year-old woman with advanced breast cancer and her son/caregiver in their home. The nurse knows this patient well but notices that on this visit the woman has not maintained eye contact with the nurse or her son. The nurse should ask

    A. The patient why she is not making eye contact.

    B. The son if his mother has a history of mental illness.

    C. The son how long his mother has been exhibiting these behaviors.

    D. To speak to the patient alone.

56. Answer is C

    A. Incorrect: It is unlikely that this degree of clutter has occurred recently since receiving a terminal diagnosis.

    B. Incorrect: This degree of clutter represents an ongoing issue most likely predating the terminal illness and any debilitation resulting from that.

    C. **Correct:** Hoarding disorder is characterized by a persistent difficulty in parting with possessions to the point of excess often resulting in extreme clutter throughout the home.

    D. Incorrect: The accumulation of this degree of clutter most likely represents an ongoing issue occurring over several years and predates the more recent terminal diagnosis.

57. Answer is A

    A. **Correct:** Patients with psychiatric diagnoses often have undertreated pain.

    B. Incorrect: There is no evidence that patients with borderline personality disorders have lower pain thresholds.

    C. Incorrect: The nurse should not assume that patients with borderline personality disorders are drug seeking without conducting a full assessment.

    D. Incorrect: Haloperidol is not an effective treatment for pain.

58. Answer is B

    A. Incorrect: Visual hallucinations are not a common symptom of neuropathic pain.

    B. **Correct:** Excessive alcohol use is often underreported by patients. Insomnia, shaking, sweating, and agitation are common signs of alcohol withdrawal.

    C. Incorrect: The presence of a fever has not been established and should, therefore, not be treated as a first action.

    D. Incorrect: Evidence that this is an emergent situation cannot be determined without additional information.

59. Answer is D

    A. Incorrect: The nurse should first ask to speak to the patient alone to ensure privacy and safety before asking if something is wrong.

    B. Incorrect: The nurse knows this patient well and sees this behavior as unusual. The nurse should not assume that a chronic mental illness is the reason for the patient's difficulty.

    C. Incorrect: Until it is determined that the patient is not autonomous, she should be interviewed directly.

    D. **Correct:** This action gives the nurse and patient privacy to talk about the nurse's observations.

60. A patient tells the nurse that he knows he will go to hell when he dies because Jesus is jealous of his powers and will not let him in heaven. The best explanation for this behavior is

    A. Alcohol withdrawal.

    B. Delusional activity.

    C. Hallucinations.

    D. Opioid toxicity.

61. During a hospice admission interview, a 67-year-old woman with advanced cardiac disease admits to being treated for depression in her 30s. The nurse understands that the patient

    A. Is at no greater risk of depression because of the time span since the original diagnosis.

    B. Should be closely monitored due to a greater risk for depression with this illness.

    C. Should be placed on prophylactic antidepressants.

    D. Should be placed on suicide watch until the risk assessment can be completed.

62. A patient has been experiencing poorly controlled neuropathic pain for several weeks, but is otherwise stable. As the nurse prepares to leave his home, he tells the nurse "I don't think I'll be here when you come back." The most appropriate question from the nurse is

    A. "Are you having premonitions that you will die soon?"

    B. "Are you angry about something?"

    C. "Are you planning a trip to see your daughter?"

    D. "Can you tell me why you think that you won't be here?"

63. The nurse providing wound care to a male patient with schizophrenia should

    A. Give report to oncoming nurses just outside of the patient's room.

    B. Tell the patient when she will touch him.

    C. Place a fan at the foot of the patient's bed to reduce hot flashes.

    D. Use only natural light in the room.

60. Answer is B

    A. Incorrect: Delusions are not a common symptom of alcohol withdrawal, although occasionally patients can experience hallucinations with alcohol withdrawal.

    B. **Correct:** Delusions are fixed, false beliefs that the patient insists are real.

    C. Incorrect: Hallucinations involve one of the senses (e.g., auditory, tactile) while the patient is fully awake.

    D. Incorrect: Delusions are not a common symptom of opioid toxicity.

61. Answer is B

    A. Incorrect: The patient may be at risk for depression as evidenced by her prior history and depending on her current support and coping mechanisms.

    B. **Correct:** The stress of the terminal illness can exacerbate the patient's tendency for depression and she should be monitored closely.

    C. Incorrect: The use of prophylactic antidepressants is not warranted and there is no evidence to support this use.

    D. Incorrect: The patient will not require suicide watch until the plan, intent, and means of self-harm are documented.

62. Answer is D

    A. Incorrect: This remark does not address the immediate safety concern of self-harm.

    B. Incorrect: There is no reason to believe that the patient is angry and this remark does not address the immediate safety concern of self-harm.

    C. Incorrect: This remark completely disregards the severity of this patient's remark and may even suggest that the nurse is unwilling to discuss the real problem.

    D. **Correct:** More information is needed as the nurse should always consider such remarks made by patients as if the patient is contemplating self-harm.

63. Answer is B

    A. Incorrect: Giving report outside of the patient's room can be perceived by the patient as whispering or talking about him behind his back.

    B. **Correct:** Nurses caring for patients with schizophrenia should avoid physical contact when possible and warn patients when they must touch them.

    C. Incorrect: Having a fan in the patient's room could be a source of injury.

    D. Incorrect: Although stimuli should be kept to a minimum, nurses must ensure that they have proper lighting to provide wound care.

Care of the Family

64. Grief expressed by family members at the time of a patient's death
    A. Indicates that the interdisciplinary team has not prepared the family for the death.
    B. Is a normal response to loss.
    C. Is a warning sign of an imminent spiritual crisis.
    D. Is usually a sign that the family is in conflict.

65. The hospice bereavement coordinator observes that after 12 months of bereavement support, a widow is expressing strong yearning for her husband, disturbing nightmares of his death, and guilt that his death was "her fault." This may suggest
    A. Alcohol misuse.
    B. Complicated grief.
    C. Disenfranchised grief.
    D. Lack of family support.

66. Carefully assessing the strengths of a family caregiver includes learning
    A. A detailed substance use history of the caregiver.
    B. Caregiver denial and reluctance to "face the facts."
    C. Caregiver history in coping with uncertainty.
    D. Why the caregiver has failed to follow through with interdisciplinary team's suggestions.

67. Puchalski's FICA is a tool for conducting a spiritual assessment. The FICA acronym stands for
    A. Faith, Influence, Community, and Address.
    B. Faith, Influence, Community, and Assessment.
    C. Follow, Interdisciplinary, Community, and Address.
    D. Follow, Interdisciplinary, Community, and Assessment.

64. Answer is B

- A. Incorrect: A family able to express grief at the time of death may indicate family safety in expressing feelings and may indicate good preparation of the family.
- B. **Correct:** Grief is a normal response to loss, especially death. Family's grief response should be validated and normalized.
- C. Incorrect: Expressions of grief are congruent in most faith traditions and do not predict spiritual crisis or spiritual well-being.
- D. Incorrect: Family members may express grief in different ways, but grief itself or varying expressions of grief do not represent conflict.

65. Answer is B

- A. Incorrect: None of the symptoms described suggest inappropriate use of alcohol.
- B. **Correct:** Yearning, intrusive thoughts and dreams, and guilt are all indicators of complicated grief more than 6 months post-loss.
- C. Incorrect: Disenfranchised grief refers to grief that is not socially endorsed.
- D. Persons with complicated grief often withdraw from existing social supports, but this does not indicate a lack of family support or unwillingness of family to offer support.

66. Answer is C

- A. Incorrect: While an important potential concern, this is not part of a strength-based assessment.
- B. Incorrect: While an important concern, this is not part of a strength-based assessment. Assessment of denial requires a thorough clinical evaluation.
- C. **Correct:** Coping style and history of coping with past challenges, particularly losses, is an important part of strength-based assessment. Strength-based assessment identifies caregiver strengths and incorporates them into the plan of care.
- D. Incorrect: While an important concern, this is not part of a strength-based assessment. The term "failed" is judgmental and is a deficit-focused view.

67. Answer is A

- A. **Correct:** Puchalski's FICA stands for Faith (what faith does individual have), Influence (how influential is this faith), Community (what faith community does individual participate in), and Address (how would individual like the interdisciplinary team to address the individual's spiritual needs).
- B. Incorrect: The A does not represent Assessment, it represents Address.
- C. Incorrect: The 'F' does not represent Follow, it represents Faith and the 'I' does not represent Interdisciplinary, it represents Influence as previously described.
- D. Incorrect: The 'F' does not represent Follow, it represents Faith and the 'I' does not represent Interdisciplinary, it represents Influence.

68. The search for ultimate meaning and purpose of life, which may involve a connection to a higher power is

   A. Faith.

   B. Religion.

   C. Religiosity.

   D. Spirituality.

69. In palliative care, the "unit of care" consists of

   A. Interdisciplinary team and family.

   B. Patient and family.

   C. Patient and interdisciplinary team.

   D. Patient and physician.

70. Comprehensive resource assessment

   A. Includes collaboration with the interdisciplinary team.

   B. Generalizes discussion of concrete resource programs.

   C. Defers to social work/case management.

   D. Is limited to a financial needs assessment.

71. Cultural humility is

   A. Apologizing for what you do not know and seeking Internet assistance.

   B. Knowing everything about the populations you serve and offering to assist colleagues.

   C. Ongoing practice of self-awareness and self-critique that addresses power imbalance inherent in medical system.

   D. Viewing culture through your own religious and family experiences.

68. Answer is D

    A. Incorrect: Faith is defined as the acceptance, without objective proof of something (e.g., God).

    B. Incorrect: Religion is defined as organized, codified, and often institutionalized beliefs and practices that express one's spirituality.

    C. Incorrect: Religiosity is defined as the quality of being religious; piety; devoutness.

    D. **Correct:** Spirituality is the broad term used to describe the search for ultimate meaning and purpose of life involving a connection to a higher power.

69. Answer is B

    A. Incorrect: The interdisciplinary team provides the care and is not part of the unit of care.

    B. **Correct:** Patient and family make up the unit of care. Providing care for the patient must include care for the family (as defined by the patient) as a singular unit.

    C. Incorrect: The interdisciplinary team provides the care and is not part of the unit of care.

    D. Incorrect: The physician is one member of the interdisciplinary team and is not part of the unit of care.

70. Answer is A

    A. **Correct:** Interdisciplinary team collaboration promotes clear understanding of specific resources available to each patient–family unit.

    B. Incorrect: Reviewing programs generally increases confusion and can mislead the patient–family unit as to their options.

    C. Incorrect: Nursing input is essential to the high-quality, whole-person care plan.

    D. Incorrect: Financial needs assessment is an important component in understanding the resources each patient and family unit needs, but it is does not provide the whole picture.

71. Answer is C

    A. Incorrect: Humility is a practice of ongoing learning. While it may include apologizing, if you make a mistake or offend a patient or family member, it is not the central practice.

    B. Incorrect: While it is necessary practice to obtain basic information about the populations you serve, this knowledge base is ever-building. You cannot know everything.

    C. **Correct:** Cultural humility is a life-long process addressing power imbalances due to race, class, gender, sexuality, nation, ability, language, etc.

    D. Incorrect: It is the professional responsibility of all clinicians to understand the influence of their own religious and family experiences in order to put them aside and work from where the patient and family are.

72. Culturally sensitive communication by the interdisciplinary team is demonstrated by

    A. Circumventing communication styles.

    B. Minimizing patient and family roles in decision-making.

    C. Team-centered interviewing strategies.

    D. Using professionally trained interpreters.

73. Before a scheduled visit to see Mrs. Alexander today, the hospice nurse has been informed that she was seen in the emergency room last night due to side effects from giving herself too much pain medication. How can the nurse assure that Mrs. Alexander understands the directions for taking her medications?

    A. Ask her husband to make sure she takes her medications correctly.

    B. Carefully explain the times and amount of each medication.

    C. Confirm understanding by using the "teach back" method.

    D. Refer her to the pharmacist of her local drugstore.

Dying Patient in Various Care Settings

74. Hospital-based palliative care programs have been shown to be advantageous because

    A. Hospitals can bill Medicare, Medicaid, and private insurance for 100% of the services offered by palliative care teams.

    B. Their location in primarily low income and rural area hospitals increases access to palliative care for these populations.

    C. They help patients and families clarify goals of care, resulting in improved pain control and symptom management, and decrease intensive care unit length of stays.

    D. They offer comfort care for patients when all other treatment options have been exhausted.

72. Answer is D

   A.   Incorrect: Each patient and family unit has unique communication styles. It is the role of the interdisciplinary team to identify these styles and utilize them to enhance communication.

   B.   Incorrect: Family roles in decision-making vary across different cultural and religious backgrounds. The team must try its best to understand these dynamics to enhance communication outcomes. For example, in some Asian families, addressing the patient's eldest son will be necessary for care planning.

   C.   Incorrect: Communication strategies should be patient- and family-centered.

   D.   **Correct:** Try to avoid using family members as translators as they interpret through their own emotional and cognitive reactions. If the patient requests family to act as interpreter after psychoeducation review's benefit of professionally-trained interpreter services, proceed with family interpretation. This may be the culturally appropriate intervention.

73. Answer is C

   A.   Incorrect: While it is valuable for another member of the family to understand correct dosing, the patient must understand since she is the one dosing herself.

   B.   Incorrect: As careful as we are in explaining dose and frequency, up to 50% of prescription and over-the-counter medications are taken incorrectly.

   C.   **Correct:** Utilizing the teach back method has proven to confirm understanding by the patient. Use an open-ended question such as "I want to be sure I have instructed you correctly. Can you explain to me how you will take this medication?"

   D.   Incorrect: The local pharmacist, while very helpful in answering questions, should not be the person to teach medication administration.

Dying Patient in Various Care Settings

74. Answer is C

   A.   Incorrect: Currently, only physician and advanced practice registered nurses' (APRN) palliative care consultations and visits can be billed to insurance companies. There is no reimbursement, other than philanthropy, for other palliative care services.

   B.   Incorrect: Low income and rural areas have the lowest numbers of palliative care hospital programs throughout the United States.

   C.   **Correct:** Recent research has demonstrated that palliative care teams in hospitals are effective in providing earlier clarification of patient/family preferences, improved levels of pain and symptom management, and shorter stays in intensive care unit (ICU) settings.

   D.   Incorrect: Palliative care services can be offered concurrently with curative treatments to enhance patient comfort and quality of life.

75. When providing hospice and palliative care to individuals with intellectual and developmental disabilities, it is important to recognize

    A. Deficits in cognition and communication may make it difficult for patients to understand their illness and verbalize their symptoms.

    B. Patients with intellectual and developmental disabilities are prohibited by law from having advance directives and do not resuscitate status.

    C. Spiritual care needs of individuals with intellectual and developmental disabilities are decreased due to their disability.

    D. While in general it is important to include patients in their palliative plans of care, it is not necessary to do so for patients with intellectual and developmental disabilities as they are not likely to understand.

76. Mr. Rodriguez, a 69-year-old Latino man diagnosed 2 years ago with metastatic lung cancer that is now in end stage, is being admitted to a hospice home care program. He is retired from a meat processing plant. Mr. Rodriguez's primary language is Spanish, he is unmarried, and lives in 1 room of an inner city boarding house that is infested with bedbugs. He does not drive. His cell phone service was recently shut off. He has no family but has relied on friends in the boarding house to help him with shopping and meals. He ambulates with a cane. Mr. Rodriguez reports his pain is 7/10 and that he cannot afford the copay for his pain medication. The nurse should immediately

    A. Admit Mr. Rodriguez to hospice, contact his physician to review the initial plan of care, and request an order for pain medication.

    B. Call Adult Protective Services to report Mr. Rodriguez's unsafe living conditions.

    C. Decline to accept Mr. Rodriguez as a patient due to the lack of a primary caregiver.

    D. Request a Spanish speaking social worker be assigned to Mr. Rodriguez's case to assist him with relocation to alternate housing.

77. Which of the following response by the nurse indicates an understanding of the Medicare Conditions of Participation criteria for general inpatient hospice care? "Mrs. Smith,

    A. The inpatient hospice team has achieved a good level of comfort for your husband. His pain has been well controlled without any medication adjustments over the past few days. However, because he has experienced a decline in his condition and may only have a few weeks left, he can stay here if you both prefer."

    B. You have been doing an amazing job caring for your husband, but I can see the toll it is taking on you. I think it would be best to transfer him to an inpatient bed for symptom management for a few days so you can get some rest to enable you to continue to care for him in the coming weeks."

    C. You have been doing an amazing job caring for your husband even though medicating him every 4 hours is exhausting. Moreover, despite the recent changes we've made with his dosing, he is still very uncomfortable. I think our best option right now is to transfer him to an inpatient bed for a few days to get his pain under control."

    D. Your husband is actively dying and may only have a few days left. We can transfer him to an inpatient bed so that you can spend these last few days at his side holding his hand without worrying about having to clean and turn him."

75. Answer is A

    A. **Correct:** Depending on the degree of disability, a patient with intellectual and developmental disabilities (IID) may have difficulty understanding their health status and may be unable to describe their symptoms. It is important to use strategies and specialized assessment tools and techniques to optimize assessment and communication with IID patients.

    B. Incorrect: Although ethical issues of autonomy and competence can make healthcare decision-making complicated and present legal barriers that differ among states, persons with IID can have advance directives including Physician/Provider/Medical Orders for Life-Sustaining Treatment (P/MOLST) and do-not-resuscitate (DNR) status.

    C. Incorrect: Studies have shown that the spiritual care needs of patients with IID are similar to that of the general population.

    D. Incorrect: Every attempt should be made to include persons with IID in the hospice/palliative plan of care. Learning how to communicate with IID individuals and collaborate with group home staff can promote optimal quality of life for these individuals.

76. Answer is A

    A. **Correct:** Pain is Mr. Rodriguez's most urgent problem. As he has elected his Medicare Hospice Benefit, he will not have to pay a copay for his medication.

    B. Incorrect: Mr. Rodriguez's living conditions may not be ideal, but this scenario presents no evidence of any immediate risk to Mr. Rodriguez's safety.

    C. Incorrect: Although Mr. Rodriguez is unmarried and has identified no family support, he is able to live independently, is a competent decision-maker, and has support from friends.

    D. Incorrect: While Mr. Rodriguez's social issues may be best served by a Spanish speaking social worker, they are not his most immediate concerns.

77. Answer is C

    A. Incorrect: General inpatient care is intended to be short-term for the purpose of managing acute episodes of uncontrolled pain or other symptoms. Once symptoms have been managed, a patient must be discharged to an appropriate level of care.

    B. Incorrect: This response indicates that the nurse may be confusing the criteria for general inpatient care with inpatient respite care.

    C. **Correct:** This response by the nurse indicates an appropriate use of general inpatient level of care.

    D. Incorrect: A patient who is actively dying, without symptoms that require skilled care, is not appropriate for general inpatient care.

78. Communication and collaboration among healthcare providers is essential to the delivery of quality hospice and palliative care because

    A. Communication and collaboration eliminate conflict among internal and external team members.

    B. Effective communication and collaboration identifies common goals for patients, saving clinicians from time-consuming documentation.

    C. Good communication fosters seamless continuity of care and improved patient outcomes.

    D. Using effective communication techniques eliminates the need for ongoing evaluation of interdisciplinary team communication processes.

79. A nursing assistant working on an inpatient palliative care unit asks the nurse how she can help with Mr. Francis' pain management. Which of the following statements would be most appropriate to say to a nursing assistant?

    A. "Ask if he would like to hear about the great catch your son made yesterday."

    B. "If you see that he is not using the patient-controlled anesthesia, remind him to press the button every so often."

    C. "Let me know when he asks for pain medication and you can take it to him."

    D. "Switch assignments so that Mr. Francis is not assigned the same nursing assistant as yesterday."

80. Offender aides working in hospice prisons

    A. Can receive time off of their sentence.

    B. Can request being an aide as their prison job.

    C. Must follow the U.S. Department of Justice regulations for prison hospice.

    D. Report being able to atone for their own offenses.

78. Answer is C

    A. Incorrect: Conflicts among collaborators are inevitable. Effective communication skills help resolve them.
    B. Incorrect: Documentation of communications provides important information about patient and team goals of care and demonstrates the collaboration that is essential to the provision of quality care.
    C. **Correct:** Improved patient outcomes and maintaining healthy provider relationships are the goals of effective communication and collaboration.
    D. Incorrect: Ongoing evaluation of interdisciplinary team (IDT) communication processes, including communication skill self-assessments, is important in maintaining positive, healthy teams.

79. Answer is A

    A. **Correct:** Distraction is an effective nonpharmacological treatment for pain and it is appropriate to ask before telling personal stories. Remind the nursing assistant to shorten the story if Mr. Francis shows signs that he only agreed to hear the story to be polite (e.g., not paying attention).
    B. Incorrect: No caregivers should tell the patient when to use patient-controlled analgesia (PCA). Patients who need reminding would most likely receive better relief from other methods of pain control.
    C. Incorrect: While it is appropriate for the nursing assistant to inform the nurse when a patient asks for pain medication, it is the responsibility of the person who prepared the medication to administer it.
    D. Incorrect: Consistency in caregivers has been shown to provide nonpharmacological pain and symptom relief.

80. Answer is D

    A. Incorrect: Volunteer offender aides are not given time off of their sentence.
    B. Incorrect: Offender aides are volunteers, which is in addition to their assigned prison job.
    C. Incorrect: The U.S. Department of Justice does not have prison hospice regulations. Hospice prisons are not subject to Medicare regulations.
    D. **Correct:** Volunteer offender aides have reported finding their own humanity and found value in being able to atone for their past offenses.

81. Mr. Paul has end stage chronic obstructive pulmonary disease with a prognosis of several months. While doing his hospice admission assessment, the nurse asks Mr. Paul if he served in the military. He replied that he retired from the U.S. Navy after serving in World War II and the Korean War. Which of the following is an accurate statement about Mr. Paul? Mr. Paul

    A. Has posttraumatic stress disorder.

    B. Is stoic and will not report pain.

    C. Has been affected by his time in the military.

    D. Will want to talk about his military service.

82. Mr. Benedict is 69 years old and has considered an alley his home for many years. Through care received at a free clinic, he has been diagnosed with late-stage lung cancer and referred to hospice. Which of the following is a challenge that the hospice nurses will face when providing care to Mr. Benedict?

    A. Finding a healthcare power of attorney.

    B. Immediate admission to a hospice inpatient facility.

    C. Completing an advance directive.

    D. Not being able to use opioid pain medications.

83. Which of the following is a characteristic that many rural dwellers share?

    A. Feeling isolated.

    B. Equate being healthy with being able to work.

    C. Prefer to receive healthcare from newcomers.

    D. Feeling invisible.

81. Answer is C

    A. Incorrect: While Veterans report posttraumatic stress disorder (PTSD) more than the general population, it cannot be assumed that Mr. Paul has PTSD.

    B. Incorrect: While many Veterans exhibit stoicism related to their military training, it cannot be assumed that Mr. Paul will not report pain.

    C. **Correct:** All Veterans have been impacted by the time they served in the military each in their own way.

    D. Incorrect: Not all Veterans want to talk about their military service. Let the Mr. Paul guide the conversation about his military service.

82. Answer is A

    A. **Correct:** It would be good for Mr. Benedict to have a healthcare power of attorney to make decisions if he cannot. If he has already chosen one, the hospice will need to ensure that they can contact him/her. If he has not chosen a healthcare power of attorney, it may be difficult to find one among the people Mr. Benedict knows and he may not have had contact with family in a long time.

    B. Incorrect: While each person is unique in their choices, most homeless people chose to die where they had been living. Living in an alley does not preclude a person from receiving hospice care.

    C. Incorrect: Even though there are high rates of substance addiction and mental illness in homeless people, it cannot be assumed that this is the case for Mr. Benedict. Everyone should be asked about their wishes, even if there is a reason he/she cannot complete an advance directive. In addition, an advance directive is not required for admission to hospice.

    D. Incorrect: Theft of any medications that can be abused or sold is a concern for homeless persons, but does not preclude them from being used. A method of safe storage of all medications will be needed.

83. Answer is B

    A. Incorrect: Despite needing to travel long distances for services such as healthcare, rural dwellers do not feel isolated.

    B. **Correct:** Health is viewed as the ability to work.

    C. Incorrect: Rural dwellers prefer to receive healthcare from insiders/old-timers.

    D. Incorrect: Rural dwellers perceive a lack of anonymity.

Advance Care Planning and Goals of Care

84. The Patient Self-Determination Act requires that hospitals accepting Medicare patients must

    A. Ask if a patient has an advance directive.

    B. Document the presence of a do not resuscitate order.

    C. Ensure that patients with terminal illnesses have an advance directive.

    D. Require patients to provide copies of their advance directives.

85. Goals of advance care planning include

    A. Completion of an advance directive.

    B. Counseling for families with opposing views.

    C. Determining values and priorities for end-of-life care.

    D. Signing a do not resuscitate order.

86. Patients with an out-of-hospital do not resuscitate order

    A. Are required to wear an identification bracelet or necklace.

    B. May revoke it at any time.

    C. Must have a do not resuscitate order written in the event of hospitalization.

    D. Will not receive any aggressive treatment.

87. The Physician Orders for Life-Sustaining Treatment (POLST) differs from a living will in that POLST

    A. Is a signed medical order by a provider.

    B. Is designed for people without a life-limiting illness.

    C. Orders are situational.

    D. Requires two physician signatures.

88. The Patient Self-Determination Act (PSDA) was passed as a result of

    A. Increasing healthcare costs.

    B. Increasing medically-related lawsuits.

    C. The Karen Ann Quinlan case.

    D. The Nancy Cruzan case.

84. Answer is A
    A. **Correct:** In addition to providing information on advance directives to staff, patients, and the community, patients are asked if they have an advance directive.
    B. Incorrect: Do not resuscitate (DNR) orders are not mentioned in the Patient Self-Determination Act.
    C. Incorrect: Patients are not required to have an advance directive.
    D. Incorrect: The law requires that the organization ask about advance directives, does not require that patients provide copies.

85. Answer is C
    A. Incorrect: Do not resuscitate (DNR) order might be a result after determining goals.
    B. Incorrect: Counseling may be indicated after discussion of goals.
    C. **Correct:** Values and priorities must be determined so that other planning/decisions can be made.
    D. Incorrect: An advance directive might be a result after determining goals.

86. Answer is B
    A. Incorrect: Although some organizations may offer bracelets or necklaces, patients are not required to wear them.
    B. **Correct:** A do not resuscitate (DNR) order may be revoked at any time.
    C. Incorrect: DNR orders should be honored by receiving facilities.
    D. Incorrect: Aggressive palliative care may be indicated.

87. Answer is A
    A. **Correct:** The Physician/Provider/Medical Orders for Life-Sustaining Treatment (POLST/MOLST) provides specific instructions/orders on several medical interventions and is signed by the provider.
    B. Incorrect: POLST/MOLST is designed for persons with life-limiting illness; living will can be initiated at any time.
    C. Incorrect: Living wills include situations in which a treatment would/would not be implemented; POLST/MOLST do not.
    D. Incorrect: POLST/MOLST only requires one provider signature; living wills do not require a provider signature.

88. Answer is D
    A. Incorrect: The law did not address healthcare costs.
    B. Incorrect: The law was not related to healthcare providers being sued.
    C. Incorrect: The Karen Quinlan case was many years earlier.
    D. **Correct:** The Patient Self-Determination Act (PSDA) was passed as a result of the Nancy Cruzan case.

89. Which of the following is true about the nurse's role in advance care planning?

    A. Complete his/her own advance directive.

    B. Initiate discussion on the first encounter with the patient.

    C. Know the prognosis for the patient.

    D. Wait until the patient is close to dying.

90. The nurse's primary role in advance care planning is to

    A. Advocate for the patient.

    B. Ensure ethics committee involvement in the process.

    C. Help settle family differences.

    D. Obtain a do not resuscitate order.

91. Barriers to completion of an advance directive include

    A. Fear of substandard care.

    B. Goals of care have already been discussed.

    C. No perceived conflict among family members.

    D. Prior experience with a dying relative.

92. In discussing advance care planning with a patient with severe chronic obstructive pulmonary disease, the nurse should

    A. Determine if patient is eligible for Medicaid.

    B. Discuss smoking history.

    C. Include discussion of intubation.

    D. Not upset the patient by discussing possible intubation.

93. A family member who is designated as the healthcare power of attorney

    A. Can sign financial documents.

    B. Makes decisions in consultation with the patient and healthcare team.

    C. Must be included in all healthcare conversations.

    D. Only makes healthcare decisions when the patient lacks capacity.

89. Answer is A

    A. **Correct:** Nurses who have already completed their own advance directives will be more comfortable discussing advance directives with patients.

    B. Incorrect: A relationship with the patient should first be established.

    C. Incorrect: Advance directives can be completed by healthy individuals and prognostication can be difficult.

    D. Incorrect: Advance directives should be completed by all, not just ill patients.

90. Answer is A

    A. **Correct:** The nurses should advocate for the patient's wishes.

    B. Incorrect: Ethics committees may not be needed.

    C. Incorrect: Family differences may not be able to be resolved.

    D. Incorrect: A do not resuscitate (DNR) order may not be indicated.

91. Answer is A

    A. **Correct:** Patients may feel care will not be provided.

    B. Incorrect: When goals of care have been discussed, patients may be more receptive to advance directive.

    C. Incorrect: Conflict within families may be a barrier.

    D. Incorrect: Prior experience with a relative may increase advance directive completion.

92. Answer is C

    A. Incorrect: Payment source is not relevant to advance care planning.

    B. Incorrect: Smoking history not relevant to advance care planning.

    C. **Correct:** Intubation is a likely end stage possibility for this disease and the patient's wishes should be discussed as part of advance care planning.

    D. Incorrect: Patients need honest information to plan effectively.

93. Answer is D

    A. Incorrect: Can only sign financial documents if they are also the financial power of attorney.

    B. Incorrect: If patient is able to voice wishes, healthcare power of attorney does not need to be involved.

    C. Incorrect: The healthcare power of attorney would only be included if the patient wanted them included, or if patient lacked capacity.

    D. **Correct:** If a patient has capacity, they still make decisions.

Care of the Patient and Family in the Final Days

94. Which symptom is unlikely to occur during the final days if it has not occurred previously?

    A. Audible respiratory secretions

    B. Dyspnea

    C. Pain

    D. Restlessness

95. Which of the following should be emphasized in teaching the family about symptoms as death nears?

    A. Determining symptoms can only be done by licensed staff.

    B. Most signs of dying are distressing to the patient.

    C. The patient's self-report is the only valid way to assess symptoms.

    D. Vocalizations are not always signs of distress.

96. In the treatment of dyspnea, what is the rationale for directing a fan to the patient's face?

    A. Creating the sensation of more air.

    B. Increasing the oxygen in the room.

    C. Stimulation of the baroreceptors.

    D. The underlying mechanism is unknown.

97. In a patient nearing death, which of the following changes in breathing requires intervention?

    A. Audible respiratory secretions

    B. Cheyne-Stokes

    C. Mandibular breathing

    D. Panting

94. Answer is C

    A. Incorrect: Audible respiratory secretions are a common and expected symptom.

    B. Incorrect: Dyspnea occurs in approximately 62% of persons as death nears.

    C. **Correct:** Pain rarely occurs as a new symptom as death nears. If it does, it signifies a new issue or problem.

    D. Incorrect: Restlessness is a common and expected symptom.

95. Answer is D

    A. Incorrect: Families are often able to determine distress through behavior and or changes in expression.

    B. Incorrect: Most signs of dying are not distressing to the patient but can be quite distressing to the family.

    C. Incorrect: As death nears, the patient is often unable to self-report; symptom distress is determined by changes in behavior.

    D. **Correct:** As death nears, vocalization may occur for other reasons besides distress.

96. Answer is C

    A. Incorrect: While the patient may be comforted by a sensation of more air, it is not the underlying mechanism.

    B. Incorrect: A fan has no way of increasing the amount of oxygen.

    C. **Correct:** The baroreceptors, when stimulated, cause bronchial dilation, which is thought to reduce dyspnea.

    D. Incorrect: See C.

97. Answer is A

    A. **Correct:** Audible respiratory secretions, while a normal symptom as death nears, requires interventions such as repositioning, discontinuation of fluids, and selected medications.

    B. Incorrect: Cheyne-Stokes breathing—periods of breathing (often shallow and/or fast) that alternate with periods of apnea—is an expected breathing pattern change as death nears and requires no intervention.

    C. Incorrect: Mandibular breathing, characterized by occasional, often deep breaths where the jaw is noted to move with periods of apnea between breaths, is an expected breathing pattern as death nears and requires no intervention.

    D. Incorrect: Panting is a late but expected breathing pattern change as death nears and requires no intervention.

98. What is the guiding principle when providing care of the body after death?

   A. First, confirm death by checking for the absence of blood pressure, pupil response, and corneal reflex.

   B. If a funeral with an open casket is planned, the body should be transferred to the mortuary within 4 hours of the death.

   C. Postmortem changes are temporary.

   D. The body should always be prepared for transfer to the mortuary.

99. Which of the following describes hypoactive delirium?

   A. Agitation

   B. Calling out

   C. Lethargy

   D. Restlessness

100. Restlessness can also occur as death nears. Which of the following medications can worsen restlessness?

   A. Atypical neuroleptics

   B. Benzodiazepines

   C. Haloperidol

   D. Opioids

101. What is the overall approach to care as the patient approaches the final days?

   A. Discontinuation of routine assessments or tests that will not alter the course of care.

   B. Determine where the patient wants to die.

   C. Assure the family that the patient will not die alone.

   D. Encourage as many visitors as possible so everyone can say goodbye.

102. A 69-year-old alert patient experiencing pain from rectal cancer is very close to death. Due to a long history of taking corticosteroids, intravenous access is not dependable. Which route would be the best option for administration of analgesics for this patient?

   A. Oral

   B. Transdermal

   C. Rectal

   D. Subcutaneous

98. Answer is C

    A. Incorrect: Rarely does the nurse need to measure blood pressure, test blinking, or corneal reflex to confirm death.

    B. Incorrect: The body should be removed within 12 hours.

    C. **Correct:** All of the postmortem changes, in particular rigor mortis, are temporary.

    D. Incorrect: Body preparation is not required and may be in violation of cultural or religious traditions.

99. Answer is C

    A. Incorrect: Agitation is characteristic of hyperactive delirium.

    B. Incorrect: Calling out is characteristic of hyperactive delirium.

    C. **Correct:** Lethargy is characteristic of hypoactive delirium.

    D. Incorrect: Restlessness is characteristic of hyperactive delirium.

100. Answer is B

    A. Incorrect: Atypical neuroleptics are an option to treat restlessness.

    B. **Correct:** Benzodiazepines can have a paradoxical effect and worsen restlessness.

    C. Incorrect: Haloperidol is a first-line drug to treat restlessness.

    D. Incorrect: Opioids are not used unless the cause of the restlessness is increased pain.

101. Answer is A

    A. **Correct:** The goals and rhythm of care shift to only things that provide comfort.

    B. Incorrect: While this may change over time, this goal should have been discussed when the patient was able to fully participate in the discussion.

    C. Incorrect: As the time of death can never be accurately predicted, this is not something the staff can promise a family.

    D. Incorrect: While this varies, large numbers of visitors are generally not advised as death nears and can be a cause of confusion and restlessness.

102. Answer is D

    A. Incorrect: Oral medications may not be consistently absorbed in patients nearing death.

    B. Incorrect: Decreased circulation and increased diaphoresis in the final days mean that transdermal medications may not be absorbed as they were earlier in the disease trajectory.

    C. Incorrect: While rectal administration is an option for some when death is near, this patient's rectal cancer prohibits rectal medications.

    D. **Correct:** Even though the subcutaneous injection will cause some discomfort, it is the best option for this patient.

103. Upon entering the home of a patient, the hospice nurse is told by the patient's husband that he thinks his wife has died. Which of the following would confirm that she has died?

    A. Eyelids slightly open with a waxy appearing skin.

    B. Lack of pulse, respiration, and blood pressure.

    C. Lack of response to stimuli.

    D. Sudden bowel and bladder incontinence.

Ethical Issues in End-of-Life Care

104. What is the ethical principle that guides a patient's right to choose or refuse therapies?

    A. Autonomy

    B. Beneficence

    C. Justice

    D. Nonmaleficence

105. An ethics of care focuses on

    A. How and why nurses care for patients and not just caregiving actions.

    B. Mandated guidelines of care established by accrediting organizations of nursing.

    C. Primarily the 4 ethical principles.

    D. Where care is provided for patients.

106. What is the first step in resolving an ethical dilemma?

    A. Evaluate the possible outcomes of these actions.

    B. Gather pertinent data.

    C. Identify possible courses of action.

    D. Identify the issue.

103. Answer is B

   A. Incorrect: Eyelids slightly open and waxy appearing skin are signs that death has occurred, but not definitive signs.

   B. **Correct:** Lack of pulse, respirations, and blood are definitive signs that death has occurred, though taking a blood pressure may not be needed.

   C. Incorrect: Complete lack of stimuli is a sign that death has occurred but needs to be accompanied by lack of pulse and respirations to assure that the person is not in a coma.

   D. Incorrect: While bowel and/or bladder incontinence is a sign that death has occurred, whether sudden or not, it could indicate that the patient's condition has worsened to the point that she no longer has control of her bowels and bladder.

Ethical Issues in End-of-Life Care

104. Answer is A

   A. **Correct:** Autonomy is the right to choose freely and is based on the individual having rights to make healthcare decisions.

   B. Incorrect: Beneficence is the obligation to do good and act for another's benefit.

   C. Incorrect: Justice is fair and equitable treatment of all persons.

   D. Incorrect: Nonmaleficence is the obligation of healthcare providers to not inflict harm.

105. Answer is A

   A. **Correct:** An ethics of care incorporates how and why nurses provide care to patients, integrating a professional moral life into professional caregiving.

   B. Incorrect: Guidelines and best practices for nursing competencies are primarily focused on specific nursing interventions.

   C. Incorrect: While the 4 ethical principles guide all medical ethics, the ethics of care specifically calls attention to the way healthcare providers interact with patients.

   D. Incorrect: Ethics of care is important regardless of setting.

106. Answer is D

   A. Incorrect: Weighing possible outcomes of actions is the final step in resolving an ethical dilemma.

   B. Incorrect: While information gathering from all members involved is important, it cannot be completed before identification of the primary issue.

   C. Incorrect: Recognizing potential courses of action comes after identifying the issue and gathering pertinent data to ensure a unique approach for the specific case.

   D. **Correct:** The first step is to identify the clinical situation causing distress among healthcare team members, patients, and/or family members.

107. The following professional resources may help inform possible courses of actions and potential outcomes from an ethical dilemma **EXCEPT**

    A. Case law.

    B. Institutional or agency policies.

    C. Patient's medical record.

    D. Position and consensus statements from professional organizations.

108. Which of the following is an instance when the truth about a patient's condition may be withheld from the patient? When

    A. A patient's daughter requests that her competent mother not be told for fear that she will lose hope.

    B. Family members strongly disagree with a patient's choice of plan of care and feel that they can make a better choice.

    C. The patient is unable to speak fluent English and a translator is unavailable.

    D. The patient states he/she does not want to be burdened with the information and requests that a family member make all decisions.

109. What is the definition of substituted judgment?

    A. A patient chooses medical treatment based on the wishes of their surrogate.

    B. A surrogate relies on known preferences of a patient to make a decision about medical care.

    C. The preferences of the surrogate are substituted for the patient's wishes.

    D. When patient preferences are unknown and the surrogate must make a decision based on what a reasonable person in a similar situation would choose.

110. How might a time-limited trial of a life-prolonging therapy (e.g., hemodialysis, hydration, mechanical ventilation) be beneficial?

    A. Allows sufficient time for families to come to a decision about withholding treatment.

    B. Court involvement would not be required to deem that the therapy is medically futile.

    C. Establishes specific criteria and timeline for achieving clinical goals of these therapies, potentially relieving emotional distress of patients and families.

    D. Is seen by the courts as a friendly alternative to withdrawal of care.

107. Answer is C

    A.   Incorrect: Case law does help inform current ethical dilemmas by providing examples of how courts have decided previous, similar cases.

    B.   Incorrect: Institutional and agency policies are important resources as they may have specific guidelines for a particular setting.

    C.   **Correct:** While the patient's medical record may help inform the medical dilemma by providing specific information, it is not a professional resource.

    D.   Incorrect: Position and consensus statements are developed to provide professional guidance and should be consulted.

108. Answer is D

    A.   Incorrect: Patients have a right to the information and trained clinicians can facilitate a conversation with mother and daughter.

    B.   Incorrect: Despite family member disagreements with patient choices, patients must still be given the option to hear the truth about their medical condition.

    C.   Incorrect: Ensuring a translator for a patient whose primary language is not English is an essential component of providing care and never an excuse to withhold pertinent medical information.

    D.   **Correct:** Patients have the right to refuse additional information about their condition and refer decision-making to a surrogate.

109. Answer is B

    A.   Incorrect: Substituted judgment is made by surrogates when the patient is determined to lack decisional capacity.

    B.   **Correct:** If a surrogate has prior knowledge about a patient's preferences, he/she can use that information and be a voice for the patient's wishes.

    C.   Incorrect: Substituted judgment is predicated upon having some prior knowledge of the patient's wishes and being able to act upon them.

    D.   Incorrect: This is the definition of "best interests," which is relevant when the surrogate has no prior knowledge of the patient's wishes.

110. Answer is C

    A.   Incorrect: While a time-limited trial may give families more time to reach consensus, the focus is on the goal of the therapy. Moreover, once begun, then withholding treatment is no longer an option.

    B.   Incorrect: While medical futility is a consideration in withholding or withdrawing care, a time-limited trial assumes that some benefit may come from the intervention.

    C.   **Correct:** A time-limited trial establishes clear goals and boundaries of continuing life-prolonging therapy, thereby helping to frame the conversation for patients and families about withdrawal of care.

    D.   Incorrect: Courts have upheld the legal right to withhold/withdraw therapies, but a time-limited trial would not be an alternative to these options and would rarely be decided by a court.

111. What is the Rule of Double Effect?
    A. Allows clinicians to give medications with the intention of ending a patient's life.
    B. Establishes that morphine given for pain may also help dyspnea.
    C. Morphine given at the end of life will have double the effect than if given in prior to the end of life.
    D. The ethical justification for actions that have positive intended effects and negative unintended but foreseen effects.

112. What is the intended effect of palliative sedation?
    A. End the life of a terminally ill patient is who is suffering one or more refractory symptoms.
    B. Relieve one or more refractory symptoms of a terminally ill patient by reducing consciousness.
    C. Sedate a patient without the consent of the patient or family.
    D. Remove the ability of a patient to eat or drink near the end of life.

113. Nurses should incorporate ethical practices into their roles by doing all of the following **EXCEPT**
    A. Be an advocate for patients and families by participating in patient and family conference.
    B. Participate on ethics committees and Institutional Review Boards when possible.
    C. Practice self-reflection.
    D. Rely on interdisciplinary colleagues to keep current with ethical and legal issues related to end-of-life care.

111. Answer is D

    A.   Incorrect: The clinician must intend only the good effect, which must outweigh the bad effect.

    B.   Incorrect: While it is true that opioids given for pain may also help treat dyspnea, this is not related to the Rule of Double Effect (RDE).

    C.   Incorrect: While opioids are often a medication given at the end of life and concerns are expressed over the RDE, the effect of the medication is not doubled.

    D.   **Correct:** This is the correct definition of the RDE.

112. Answer is B

    A.   Incorrect: The intent must always be to relieve symptoms and not to end a patient's life.

    B.   **Correct:** This is the goal of palliative sedation—to relieve refractory symptoms in a terminally ill patient even when it means the patient may have reduced consciousness.

    C.   Incorrect: Palliative sedation can only be initiated with the consent of a patient or surrogate.

    D.   Incorrect: Discussions about hydration and nutrition should be separate from relief of symptoms requiring palliative sedation. Additionally, the intent of palliative sedation is never to cause more harm.

113. Answer is D

    A.   Incorrect: Advocacy is a very significant component of ethical nursing practice in end-of-life care.

    B.   Incorrect: Opportunities to serve on ethics committees and Institutional Review Boards (IRBs) are important ways to promote an ethical practice.

    C.   Incorrect: Self-reflection (being aware of one's own values, beliefs, and responses toward patients, families, and colleagues) is a principal way to foster an ethical nursing role.

    D.   **Correct:** While interdisciplinary colleagues should keep up with current issues, nurses are responsible for their own professional development for end-of-life ethical and legal issues.

Case Studies for Discussion and Answers

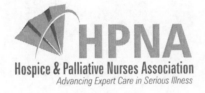

Case Study #1

A palliative care consult was requested for a 38-year-old man with colon cancer who has been receiving treatment and has been admitted to the hospital due to pain, dehydration, and anorexia. There is some suspicion that he was not taking his morphine tablets as prescribed at home. His family members are disgruntled with his pain control, weight loss, and lack of interest in food. The patient wants to continue with treatment but also wants "someone to do better" in managing these symptoms.

When the nurse arrives to initiate the consultation, several family members are present and immediately state, "We want his cancer treatment to continue and his horrible symptoms to get better. We are not familiar with *palliative care,* but some friends told us that really means *hospice*. So what are you going to do for him?"

1. What are the misconceptions?

2. How can the nurse best explain the relationship of hospice and palliative care?

3. What can the nurse say about his treatments?

4. What would be a clear statement of the goals of treatment?

The case study answers are just one possibility. You may have others.

1. **Answer:** Palliative care is often mistaken to mean hospice. The public may not understand that palliative care can be started in conjunction with curative treatment.

2. **Answer:** The Hospice and Palliative Nurses Association endorses the exact definition of palliative care originating from the National Consensus Project for Quality Palliative Care (NCP), which states: "Palliative Care means patient- and family-centered care that optimizes quality of life by anticipating, preventing, and treating suffering. Palliative care throughout the continuum of illness involves addressing the physical, intellectual, emotional, social, and spiritual needs and [facilitating] patient autonomy, access to information, and choice." The National Consensus Project further explains, "Palliative care is operationalized through effective management of pain and other distressing symptoms, while incorporating psychosocial and spiritual care with consideration of patient/family needs, preferences, values, beliefs, and culture. Evaluation and treatment should be comprehensive and patient-centered with a focus on the central role of the family unit in decision-making. Palliative care affirms life by supporting the patient and family's goals for the future, including their hopes for cure or life-prolongation, as well as their hopes for peace and dignity throughout the course of illness, the dying process, and death" (NCP, 2013, p. 9).

    The realm of palliative care services is individualized to the patient and family, occurring in the context of the diagnosis and time of initiation of services. Palliative care includes supportive counseling services, pain and symptom management, discharge planning, hospice care, and bereavement services after death. Palliative care may begin at the time of diagnosis and can be delivered simultaneously with life-prolonging therapies, during all phases of illness. Hospice care is palliative care delivered at the end of life, and in the United States is defined by the Hospice Medicare Benefit for persons with a prognosis of 6 months or less should the illness run its natural course.

3. **Answer:** His treatments will continue and, with management of his distressing symptoms, the benefits of those treatments may be enhanced.

4. **Answer:** Our goal will be to involve professional team members to address physical, emotional, and spiritual problems to provide *quality of life* as you and your family would define it, while his treatments continue.

Case Study #2

Gina is a 29-year-old with end stage cancer. As she cannot care for herself at home and neither of her divorced parents are able to care for her in their homes, she has been admitted to an inpatient hospice unit for the past 2 weeks. The main team that is caring for her consists of a physician, nurse, social worker, counselor, and chaplain who meet regularly to coordinate Gina's care. Gina is invited but refuses to go to the care meeting.

Today's team meeting has become very tense between several team members and Gina's parents, who are in attendance. It is discovered that 1 team member has been led to believe by Gina that her mother is the only one who cares about her. While another was told that only Gina's father cares about her.

1. What type of team is caring for Gina?

2. What type of behavior has Gina been exhibiting by giving different team members different information about her parents?

3. One week after the open discussion with Gina's parents, they both feel that they can take her home with hospice. They are meeting again with Gina to determine which parent will be best able to care for her, though both have agreed to support each other. Several hours before the meeting 1 of the team members, still not convinced that Gina's mother is being truthful, attempts to sway Gina into moving in with her father by telling Gina that her mother will not be physically able to care for her at home and will impose her religious beliefs on Gina. What type of boundary has this team member crossed?

4. Gina's, father who will be supporting his ex-wife as Gina moves into her mother's home, comes to you with a number of Web pages that he has printed about Gina's cancer and possibilities of a cure. What are some guidelines you can give him about gauging the trustworthiness of a website?

Case Studies for Discussion and Answers • 63

1. **Answer**: Gina is being cared for by an interdisciplinary team. An interdisciplinary team has a collaborative approach to communication and function.

2. **Answer**: Gina is exhibiting splitting—manipulating team members into choosing sides.

3. **Answer**: The team member has used deception to coerce the patient by lying about the mother.

4. **Answer**: Avoid Internet information that does not have a publisher or author; is primarily interested in selling a product; does not have a date of publication or is more than 5 years old; and claims "cures" or "miracles."

Case Study # 3

Ms. Pacelli, a 49-year-old woman, presents to the emergency department with shortness of breath. She has a history of chronic obstructive pulmonary disease (COPD) and diabetes mellitus. Her spouse reports that she has been confined to the bed for more than half of the day and uses a wheelchair when outside of the house. She is diagnosed with a pleural effusion and a lung mass on chest x-ray. A computed tomography (CT) scan confirms the lung mass is suspicious for malignancy. The patient is admitted and over the next week a series of diagnostic studies are performed. A thoracentesis is done as well and is positive for stage IV non-small cell lung cancer, the most advanced stage. A flexible bronchoscopy is done and biopsies of the lung mass and mediastinal lymph nodes reveal metastatic non-small lung cancer.

Throughout this process, the patient declines quickly and has increased pain in her chest and hips, vision changes, and headaches. Based on her new diagnoses, distress, and rapid decline, a palliative care consultation is obtained.

1. What factors are important in determining her plan of care? Who should be involved in the decision-making?

2. What associated symptoms of lung cancer should be expected?

3. The decision has been made to start radiation therapy for Ms. Pacelli. She asks when she will start to have side effects from the radiation.

4. As Ms. Pacelli's lung cancer progresses, what are the most likely sites to watch for additional metastasis?

1. **Answer:** Factors include—options for disease-specific treatment (to be determined by the oncology team), her goals of care, disposition options, and willingness to treat symptoms. It is up to Ms. Pacelli to determine who is involved in decision-making. Her physician, oncology team, palliative care team, and family of her choosing will most likely be involved.

2. **Answer:** Common associated symptoms of lung cancer include chest pain, fatigue, cough, shortness of breath, and anorexia with weight loss.

3. **Answer:** Explain that side effects can be acute, subacute, and/or late. Acute side effects are short-term and typically resolve at the conclusion of treatment. Subacute side effects appear within weeks to a few months after completion of treatment. Late side effects can occur after 6 months following treatment.

4. **Answer:** Brain, liver, bone, and adrenal glands are the most common sites of lung cancer metastasis.

Case Study #4

Mr. Leo is a 65-year-old Vietnam War Veteran with a long history of chronic illness. He has hepatitis C, hepatic cirrhosis, and chronic obstructive pulmonary disease (COPD). He states he has smoked 2 packs of cigarettes per day for the past 45 years. He denies current alcohol use or other substance misuse.

Symptoms include shortness of breath with minimal exertion, productive cough, ascites, and jaundice. He is requesting palliative care to manage his symptoms of anxiety, depression, and spiritual despair.

1. What assessments would be most significant for the palliative care nurse?

2. What questions would you like to ask for more information?

3. On medication review, what medications would you expect to see?

4. What symptoms would prompt you to consider a hospice consult?

1. **Answer:** Begin with a physical assessment of his respiratory system, determine if ascites is impacting his respiratory distress, and whether nausea or constipation is present. Ask sensitively about discomfort as Veterans may not usually voice or demonstrate pain. Perhaps unresolved symptoms are leading to the psychosocial and spiritual difficulties.

2. **Answer:** When do you feel most anxious? What spiritual activities do you pursue? What were some of your interests before you became ill, and what are you no longer able to do? What are your goals for the near future? Can I ask you some questions about your military career? I would like for our social worker and chaplain to visit with you. How do you feel about that? Consider suicidal ideation or plans.

3. **Answer:** Spironolactone for the ascites. Review his medications to determine if he is on medications for pain, anxiety, depression, constipation, or any antibiotics. After reviewing medications and discussing options with him, call the physician for further direction and orders. It is important to know if he has had a paracentesis.

4. **Answer:** If the shortness of breath continues at rest, ascites is not improved with medication, and weight loss continues at 10% or more over time, a hospice consult may be in order provided this is within the patient's goals. Hospice eligibility for liver disease includes prothrombin time prolonged to more than 5 seconds and albumin less than 2.5 mg/dL as well as his ascites.

Case Study #5

Mr. Williams is a 68-year-old Vietnam War Veteran who was diagnosed with non-small cell lung cancer 9 months ago. He has undergone several different regimens of chemotherapy along with radiation therapy. At first, this allowed him to function well but in the past 2 months, he has been losing weight and spending more than 50% of the day lying in bed or on the couch.

    He describes aching, well-localized low back pain with radiation to left leg; the pain in the leg is burning and electrical. The pain is moderate (4–5/10) at rest but becomes severe (8/10) when he stands for longer periods or when he twists (e.g., getting up out of bed or into the car). He also has pain on the right rib at the mid-thoracic level. This is throbbing and he cannot sleep on his right side; it worsens when he takes a deep breath. Imaging reveals bone metastases at L2 and the 8th rib. He is currently taking hydrocodone/acetaminophen 10 mg/325 mg 8–10/day. He states it only "takes the edge off" the pain; he denies sedation, nausea, or other adverse effects. He admits to having hard stools every 4 to 5 days and can only evacuate with straining. He is eating but reports having little appetite. He cannot sleep through the night as he is awakened by pain.

    Mr. Williams has been married for 38 years; he and his wife have 2 adult sons with 3 grandchildren. He smoked 1 to 2 packs per day for 50 years; drank 4 to 6 beers/day before cancer diagnosis but cannot stand the taste of alcohol since treatment; admits to having used marijuana as a young man and heroin in Vietnam but stopped when he returned stateside; he wonders if his grandfather was an alcoholic and states one son is in Alcoholics Anonymous (AA).

1. What type(s) of pain is Mr. Williams experiencing?

2. Devise a comprehensive analgesic plan and include medications, doses, routes of administration, and frequencies.

3. Suggest a plan to prevent or treat adverse effects of analgesics.

4. Discuss family and cultural issues that may affect the pain experience.

1. **Answer:** Mr. Williams has both nociceptive (aching back pain) and neuropathic (radiating pain to his leg that is burning and electrical) pain. He also has constant pain as well as incidental breakthrough pain (pain worsened by twisting, deep breathing).

2. **Answer:** Mr. Williams is currently taking immediate-release hydrocodone/acetaminophen that is limited by the acetaminophen content. This is also not providing constant relief through the night, nor is the relief sufficient immediately after dosing. Eight to 10 tablets of 10 mg hydrocodone is approximately equal to 80–100 mg of oral morphine. One suggestion would be to start morphine extended release 30 mg every 12 hours (60 mg/day, which is a reduction of at least 25% to account for incomplete cross-tolerance); this would be supplemented with morphine immediate release 15 mg (about 20% of the 24 hour daily dose) by mouth every 2 hours as needed. One might think about adding an adjuvant analgesic for the neuropathic pain. Gabapentin (300 mg at night for 2–3 nights, then increased to twice a day for 2–3 days, then titrated to 3 times a day) can be helpful for neuropathic pain. Slow upward titration prevents dizziness. This might be added after establishing safety and efficacy of the oral morphine.

3. **Answer:** Establish a regular bowel regimen that incorporates senna/docusate titrated to produce a soft, formed bowel movement every day or every other day.

4. **Answer:** As a Veteran, Mr. Williams may be at risk for posttraumatic stress disorder (PTSD) or other unresolved emotional responses to serving in the military that are now raised with a life-threatening illness. Issues related to substance abuse, given his past history, should be monitored. As 2 other members of his family have problems with alcohol use, family support may be needed.

Case Study #6

The wife of a 78-year-old with advanced heart failure is worried about her husband's increased dyspnea and periods of altered mental status over the past 2 days. He is still eating and drinking and there are no recent changes in his medications. He requires 1-person assistance to ambulate. On assessment, he is afebrile, bilateral rales, bilateral 2+ lower extremity edema, oriented to person and place, and denies dyspnea at rest. Both the patient and his wife are aware that his heart failure is incurable and they are hoping to keep him comfortable at home.

1. What additional questions do you want to ask as part of your assessment?

2. What are some potential causes for the altered mental status?

3. What are some interventions for his dyspnea?

4. How can you educate and prepare the patient and family for what to expect as his heart failure worsens?

1. **Answer:** The nurse should ask questions about his heart failure management. Is he taking all of his heart medications and diuretics as prescribed? Is he on a fluid or salt restriction of any kind and does he weigh himself? If ordered, is he using his oxygen appropriately? Dyspnea is a subjective symptom, the nurse should clarify with the patient when is he dyspneic. Assess the patient's level of anxiety and distress.

2. **Answer:** The nurse would explore possible causes for his altered mental status including any new medications; nicotine or alcohol withdrawal; any recent labs (check for metabolic disturbances such as hypocalcemia/hypercalcemia, renal and liver function, etc.); fever or signs of infection; and nutritional deficiencies.
   Nurse would also assess for the onset of his altered mental status; use a delirium assessment scale; and a mental status exam. Even though patient's wife said there were no recent medication changes, the nurse should do a complete medication review, pain assessment, and pulse oximetry.

3. **Answer:** If the patient is taking his medications as prescribed, the nurse should contact the provider to discuss increasing his diuretics. If the patient has morphine ordered, educate the patient and family on its use; an order for morphine should be requested if they do not have one. He may benefit from an increase in the oxygen liter flow and use of a fan along with relaxation strategies if he becomes anxious. Inhalers are helpful for wheezing so in this case are not likely to be of any benefit. Leg elevation, diuretics, and compression hose may help the leg edema.

4. **Answer:** The patient and his wife have expressed comfort goals and should be asked what they know about home hospice support. The hospice agency will often send out a nurse and social worker to discuss hospice with them. Many patients and families worry about how their symptoms will be managed in the dying process. They should be asked if this is something of concern and do they want to discuss the dying process and what to expect. Education about management of respiratory symptoms should focus on strategies to maintain comfort, including morphine or opioids as needed along with medications to manage anxiety and delirium.

Case Study #7

You are admitting a 36-year-old man with stage IV liver and pancreatic cancer who has a history of alcoholism and prescription medication abuse. He is estranged from his wife and 10-year-old son due to spousal abuse.

1. What immediate assessment data should you gather in regard to his drug and alcohol issues?

2. What interventions do you need to do to set up adequate pain management for this patient?

3. What nonpharmacological therapies should the nurse consider in this situation?

4. Describe how the interdisciplinary team can be involved with this patient's care.

1. **Answer:** How long has he been drinking and taking drugs? How long has it been since his last drink and/or last medication? What types of alcohol and drugs did he abuse? How much alcohol/drugs does he take in a 24-hour period? Who does he presently have as a support system? Who is his healthcare surrogate if he has one?

2. **Answer:** Written contract for compliance, use of adjuvants, lock box, and/or daily delivery, random urine tests, and use long-acting round the clock pain medications.

3. **Answer:** Relaxation therapy, distraction, and journaling.

4. **Answer:** Be consistent in approach; determine the extent that his family may or may not want to be involved; work with patient on his feelings about his relationship with his family; provide support for the patient; ensure that family has bereavement and psychosocial support.

Case Study #8

You are caring for a 56-year-old man with end-stage chronic obstructive pulmonary disease (COPD) and schizophrenia who is addicted to tobacco. He lives with his borderline personality sister who is periodically incarcerated. His sister is his healthcare surrogate.

The patient periodically turns and looks like he is listening to someone. He has the blinds pulled and whispers when he talks to you. He believes that he is being watched by the news crew on television and that they steal his thoughts. His grooming and self-care is poor. He continues to smoke, even though there is oxygen in the home.

1. What symptoms would indicate that the patient has schizophrenia?

2. What are 3 top priority issues for dealing with this patient situation?

3. What medications are commonly used to treat the symptoms of schizophrenia?

4. What are some strategies of dealing with a borderline personality healthcare surrogate?

1. **Answer:** Blinds pulled, whispering, delusional ideas of reference, auditory/visual hallucinations.

2. **Answer:** Smoking with oxygen; finding out if the voices he hears are command voices; a possibly inappropriate healthcare surrogate.

3. **Answer:** Haloperidol, chlorpromazine, perphenazine, fluphenazine.

4. **Answer:** Observe behavior and establish a trusting relationship by showing interest and empathy; secure verbal or written contracts against violence to self or others; role model appropriate expression of feeling; encourage communications about feelings; increase team communication and consistency to prevent splitting; redirect unacceptable behaviors into acceptable outlets such as exercise or meditation; whenever conversing maintain attitude of "it is not you, but your behavior that is unacceptable."

Case Study #9

Ms. Clement, a 52-year-old African-American, recently retired, single woman, was admitted to the hospital with sudden onset of dyspnea at rest, profound weakness, syncope, and fatigue. She has a long-standing history of heart failure with repeated admissions and is nonadherent with medications (i.e., vasodilators, diuretics, and antidepressants). Ejection fraction is < 20%, Palliative Performance status = 50. Limited family support provided by elderly parents who are in poor health, 3 siblings, and a few nieces who are here when the patient is in an acute crisis but disappear once she is discharged from the hospital. Her father is a retired pastor of the African-American Methodist Episcopal Church. Ms. Clement lives alone on the 3rd floor of an apartment complex without elevators. No official healthcare proxy has been named and code status has not been addressed. She states she "makes decisions with her family and God." Family goals are to ensure "patient receives everything medicine has to offer." Patient stated goal is to "keep me out of the hospital with God's help." Family is stressed by patient's increasing symptoms and physician's recent recommendation to consider hospice care now that she is eligible. Family seems to distrust medical professionals knowing she has been ill like this before and has "bounced back."

1. What might the ethnic and cultural concerns be in this case?

2. Given the spiritual supports that Ms. Clements has identified, how would you and your team join the patient in approaching advance care planning conversations?

3. What resources and support would this patient need to meet her goal of staying at home and not in the hospital?

4. Recognizing the patient and family as the unit of care and the family's apprehension, how would you and your team approach the goals of care discussions?

1. **Answer**: Ethnic and cultural concerns include the historic distrust among some African-Americans in terms of access to medical care. The recommendation to refer this patient to hospice may generate distrust. Hospice has been underutilized by African-Americans, and may be interpreted as "giving up" the goal of cure and withholding the aggressive care this family has requested.

2. **Answer**: This patient having been raised in a very religious family, has described her decision-making as with "family and God," and her main goal is to "keep me out of the hospital with God's help." These repeated expressions firmly support her spiritual strengths. It is recommended to use FICA or SPIRIT as your spiritual assessment tool to obtain the necessary information to guide the advance care planning conversations. A referral to the palliative care chaplain would be helpful to offer additional interpretation and support for this patient and collaborate with the patient's personal spiritual counselor for ongoing spiritual support.

3. **Answer**: Concerns for the location of this patient's living quarters, the reasons for nonadherence of the medication regime, the symptoms of weakness and fatigue that plague this patient, and the limited support available to a patient basically confined to bed creates multiple areas of need to ensure she can remain in her home as is her wish. Suggestions for interventions include

    a. Contacting local support agencies such as Area Agency on Aging, Meals on Wheels, etc.
    b. Requesting home health follow-up if patient/family decline hospice.
    c. Hospice services if patient/family agree—seeking volunteer services through hospice.
    d. Safety checks for the home in terms of bathroom safety, smoke alarms, area rugs, etc.
    e. Durable medical equipment to assist with activities of daily living such as bedside commode, assistive devices, chair lifts, etc.
    f. Conversations with family members and friends chosen by patient to develop a schedule of support and assistance.
    g. Rearrangement within living quarters (first floor, preferably no steps).
    h. Enlist support of church community, as patient wishes.
    i. Explore availability to a computer and access to Internet connections and possibility for online support services.

4. **Answer**: Identifying nonadherence as a major contributor to re-hospitalizations due to uncontrolled heart failure, goals of care discussions must include exploration of reasons for nonadherence. Areas to explore include financial concerns, physical exhaustion resulting in inability to prepare her own medications, forgetfulness, depression, desire for socialization secondary to loneliness, and inability to refill prescriptions. The patient has expressed her desire to stay at home; therefore, the conversation must include educating her about her physical condition and progression of illness. Concerns expressed by the family regarding the recommendation for hospice should be addressed in a positive way, emphasizing symptom management and potential to accomplish life goals. Explaining the cause of the symptoms relative to the low ejection fraction as well as describing the weakening heart is necessary to educate the patient and family. Focusing and directing every aspect of the conversation on the patient's wish to remain at home is the single most important goal. Fostering hope, respecting the patient and family's views, and validating their concerns facilitates timely and effective transition to the next setting of care (home health, hospice, or continued reliance on informal support).

Case Study #10

Mrs. John, a 96-year-old widow, has been receiving home palliative care following a stroke that affected her right leg. She is ambulatory with a cane except for stairs, has no cognitive deficits, and can do her activities of daily living, but not her instrumental activities of daily living. Her son and daughter, who are both in their 70s, live nearby, but are not able to care for their mother in their homes. Mrs. John has chosen to move to a long-term care facility.

1. What type of long-term care facility would be best suited to meet Mrs. John's needs?

2. The home palliative care nurse (who will follow Mrs. John in the long-term care facility) visits Mrs. John on the morning of her move to the long-term care facility. Mrs. John's daughter is there and is very tearful. She is regretting the decision to let "strangers take care of her mother." How would the nurse best assist the daughter with her mother's transition to the long-term care facility?

3. What measures can the nurses at the long-term care facility put in place to prevent unnecessary transfers to the hospital for Mrs. John?

4. Though they have had residents receive hospice care, this is the first time that a resident in this long-term care facility has received care from a palliative care nurse. The long-term care facility nurses are asking what the difference is between hospice and palliative care.

1. **Answer**: As Mrs. John does not need assistance with her physical care or 24-hour nursing care, assisted living would allow her to remain relatively independent while providing meals, housekeeping, and laundry assistance.

2. **Answer**: The decision to admit a loved one to a long-term care facility is difficult for family members. They often have feelings of guilt or abandonment due to inability to care for a loved one and do not want to give up caregiving activities. Mrs. John will most likely have difficulties related to loss of her independence, loss of her home, living in a strange place, and new routines. Support for residents and families includes providing emotional support by acknowledging the difficulty of this transition and information about the facility (e.g., the level of care provided, meal times, visiting hours, activities that involve family).

3. **Answer**: By knowing common reasons for hospital admissions, measures can be put in place to prevent them. The most common clinical reasons for hospital transfers include septicemia, pneumonia, congestive heart failure, urinary tract infections, and aspiration pneumonia. Additional risks for hospitalization or rehospitalization include recent hospitalization, hypercarbia in residents with chronic obstructive pulmonary disease (COPD), poor renal function, clinical instability, and depression. For the common nonclinical reasons (e.g., availability and training of nursing home staff, physician availability), further education and putting policies in place are needed. Advance directives are also important to prevent hospital transfers for residents who do not want to be hospitalized. Fall risk precautions need to be put in place. Lower rates of hospital readmission have been seen with consistent geriatric assessment and nurse practitioner involvement.

4. **Answer**: Palliative care means patient- and family-centered care that optimizes quality of life by anticipating, preventing, and treating suffering. Palliative care throughout the continuum of illness involves addressing physical, intellectual, emotional, social, and spiritual needs and facilitating patient autonomy, access to information, and choice. Hospice care is palliative care. In the United States, hospice is largely defined by the Medicare Hospice Benefit, which places hospice care at the last 6 months of a person's life should the illness run its natural course. While palliative care is not directly paid for, hospice is paid for through the Medicare Hospice Benefit, Medicaid, Veterans Administration, and private insurance.

Case Study #11

A 78-year-old patient with severe chronic obstructive pulmonary disease (COPD) talks with you about her desire not to go back to the hospital. She states she is tired of all the "poking and sticking" and wants no more tubes. She wants to spend time with her beloved 12-year-old cocker spaniel, sleep in her own bed, and be comfortable. She is cared for by her 50-year-old son, who lives with her, and has a daughter out of state who is her financial power of attorney. She reports that her daughter is upset that she is "giving up" and has contacted her mother's pastor to have him talk with her about the need to "do everything" and leave the final decisions "in God's hands." Her son understands his mother's wish not to go back to the hospital, and feels that his sister does not understand how weak and uncomfortable their mother has become. The patient currently does not have any advance directives, physician orders for life-sustaining treatment (POLST, which are legal in her state), or a do not resuscitate order.

1. What are this patient's goals of care?

2. What steps might be taken to assist her in meeting her goals of care?

3. Who should be included in discussing her advance care planning?

4. What issues should be discussed as part of her advance care planning?

1. **Answer:** Wants to stay home, out of hospital with her dog. No more "poking," "sticking," and "tubes." Clarification is needed to know what she specifically does not want (e.g., IVs, blood draws, intubation). She wants to be comfortable, which also needs clarification to determine what this means to her.

2. **Answer:** Obtain additional information to clarify goals. Discuss possibility of completing an advance directive, physician orders for life-sustaining treatment (POLST), and a do not resuscitate (DNR) order depending on her goals of care. Discuss who she would want to be her decision-maker if she is unable to make her own healthcare decisions. Clarify with patient and son that her daughter's power of attorney is only for financial decisions unless healthcare issues are specifically addressed. Offer to have a conversation via telephone or video with her daughter to address any concerns.

3. **Answer:** Ideally, the patient should include her daughter and son in discussions, but it is up to her as to who is included. The nurse may offer to assist in answering questions and advocating for the patient. May also consider talking with pastor if this is an influential person in their lives.

4. **Answer:** Need clarification of what care she wants and does not want. Should discuss wishes regarding resuscitation/intubation. Discuss potential risks/benefits of resuscitation/intubation, as well as artificial hydration/nutrition and antibiotics. Is she eligible for hospice care? Hospice may reduce some of the caregiving burden on her son.

Case Study #12

Mr. Hank Marks, 85 years old, is admitted to your palliative care unit after a fall in his home yesterday. Due to a massive subdural hematoma and poor prognosis, his family has agreed to keep him comfortable and not prolong his life. This is in keeping with his advance directive and wishes. He was extubated in the emergency room and is unresponsive, but moaning and thrashing his arms and legs. He is accompanied to the unit by his wife of 60 years, Mary, and their daughter Margaret. The emergency department nurse also reports to you:

- History of smoking—30-pack-years.
- History of alcohol abuse. Mary and Margaret report that he hasn't been drinking for the past several years and was not drunk at the time of the fall.
- Vital signs—blood pressure, 110/60 mm Hg; pulse, 78 bpm; respirations, 40 per minute

Mary and Margaret are shaken and report feeling "numb." Margaret called her brother Mike who lives on the other side of the country but he is not able to come immediately due to a storm.

1. What are your first priorities in caring for the Marks family?

2. You suspect Mr. Marks may have developed either delirium or restlessness. What are possible underlying causes?

3. The Marks family is sitting at the bedside and is uncertain about what to do. How can you involve them in Mr. Marks' care?

4. Later in the day, you notice Mr. Marks' breathing has changed, his extremities are cooler, and he is diaphoretic. Which signs and symptoms should you be especially alert for?

1. **Answer:** Provide comfort to the patient (i.e., control symptoms), facilitate open and honest communication with the family, role model slowed pace, gentle touch, confirm the goals of care, provide anticipatory guidance, allow for emotional expression, normalize the dying process, providing privacy, assess for any religious or cultural needs.

2. **Answer:** The most likely causes of delirium and/or restlessness in Mr. Marks are nicotine withdrawal, dyspnea, urinary retention, pain, or constipation. Alcohol withdrawal is not likely a cause in this case.

3. **Answer:** Model talking to him, noting that even though he is not able to respond, he might be able to hear them. Encourage touch, music, foot or hand rubs. If appropriate, Mary might want to lie down next to him in bed or Mike may want to talk to his father by phone or video chat.

4. **Answer:** Audible respiratory secretions, restlessness, increased temperature, dyspnea, and pain can be distressing symptoms at the end of life and should be treated.

Case Study #13

Mrs. Allen is an 85-year-old patient with metastatic breast cancer and lives with her daughter, Laura. She is experiencing severe, refractory pain to her back, right shoulder, and right hip. Her opioids have been titrated up appropriately, but despite these efforts, she is suffering greatly. She also has brain metastases making her occasionally confused, although she is still able to have coherent conversations. During your visit, Laura asks to speak with you privately from her mother. She tells you that her mother has stopped eating in order to end her life because her suffering is so great and she feels as though her life is not worth living. Laura expresses that she is not ready to let go of her mother yet and hopes that her symptoms will just go away. Additionally, they do not live in a state that allows for assisted suicide.

1. How would you respond to Laura initially? What ethical principle(s) are involved?

2. What are some additional considerations for approaching this case?

3. Who might you consider involving in this case?

4. What is the nurse's role in this situation?

1. **Answer:** Providing compassionate presence in what is obviously a clear ethical dilemma for this family is paramount. Understanding the clinical issues and then collecting additional information from the patient, family members, and clinical documentation become important to help Laura and her mother develop a care plan that addresses the seriousness of her symptoms and quality of life issues. The principle of autonomy is significant in this case because of Mrs. Allen's right to choose or refuse treatments.

2. **Answer:** Escalating symptoms that have now become refractory might require consideration of palliative sedation. Symptom management guidelines and determination of decisional capacity might be important—does Mrs. Allen fully understand the risks and benefits of withholding nutrition?

3. **Answer:** When a patient has refractory symptoms and is requesting assisted suicide, it is imperative to involve the entire interdisciplinary team. A full assessment by each member might help address the symptom as well as the feelings of despair. The ethics committee at the agency may also be of assistance if conflict continues among the patient, family members, and healthcare staff.

4. **Answer:** The nurse's role includes being competent in symptom management in order to provide the best clinical care according to current guidelines. The nurse also must be in a position to advocate for Mrs. Allen and Laura as they are both seeking additional care. Advocacy in this case might mean presenting the case to the interdisciplinary team (as noted above), and ensuring that appropriate advance care planning documents are completed so that Laura may use substituted judgment if her mother becomes incapacitated as a medical decision-maker.

Pharmacology Study Questions and Answers

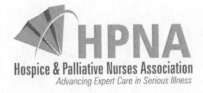

Medication Questions

1. Mrs. Como states "I know my husband is in a lot of pain from his cancer, but I'm not going to give him the oxycodone and let him get addicted." How would you respond to Mrs. Como?

2. Why can the dose of morphine be increased multiple times as needed, but the dose of acetaminophen cannot be increased beyond a certain dose?

3. How does high-dose opioid therapy cause myoclonus?

4. Which is the best opioid for relief of dyspnea?

5. When used to prevent a partial bowel obstruction from becoming complete, by what routes and doses can octreotide be given?

6. What are the considerations when selecting a medication for insomnia?

7. What are some of the challenges presented when using warfarin for patients who are debilitated?

1. **Answer:** Addiction is characterized by behaviors like not being able to control the amount of drug that a person takes, using it even when there is no pain, and continued use despite harm. We know Mr. Como has pain so this does not apply to him. The pain medication will not only decrease his pain, but once his pain is controlled, he will most likely have a better quality of life by participating in activities with you and the rest of your family.

2. **Answer:** Analgesic ceiling is the highest safe dose of a medication. Acetaminophen has a recommended ceiling dose due to the potential to compromise hepatic and renal function. Pure opioids do not have a specific ceiling dose, though doses could be limited due to active metabolites. Note that opioid doses must be titrated up slowly.

3. **Answer:** High-dose opioid therapy has the potential to cause myoclonus due to increased levels of 3-glucuronide opioid metabolites, which are the most likely cause of the neuro-excitatory side effects.

4. **Answer:** All opioids work similarly. It is not necessary to use morphine if taking another opioid for pain.

5. **Answer:** Octreotide can be given subcutaneously (100–300 mcg 2–3 times/day), continuous intravenous or subcutaneous infusion (10–40 mcg/hour), or intramuscular depot injection (20 mg intragluteally every 4 weeks once stabilized on intravenous/subcutaneous for at least 2 weeks). Octreotide cannot be given orally.

6. **Answer:**
   - Should be used in conjunction with nonpharmacological interventions.
   - Benefits must be balanced against the risk of interaction among other medications.
   - Consider both short- and long-acting sleep aids.
   - Nonbenzodiazepines are generally better tolerated and more effective than benzodiazepine medications. There is reduced dependency, reduced rebound insomnia, and a reduced tendency for drowsiness upon awakening.
   - Benzodiazepines can be used to aid in anxiety; not effective with continuous use.
   - Antihistamines are used for seasonal allergies, but have the effect of making someone sleepy.
   - Some antidepressants may have some added benefit of improving sleep.

7. **Answer:**
   - Difficult to manage in patients with poor oral intake.
   - Monitoring requires frequent venipunctures.

8. What is the limit on the amount of acetaminophen a person should receive per day?

9. What are the teaching points for lidocaine patches?

10. What are extrapyramidal symptoms? Why is it important to assess for extrapyramidal symptoms? Which medications have a high potential to cause extrapyramidal symptoms?

11. Guaifenesin is a(n)
    A. Antibiotic.
    B. Antitussive.
    C. Expectorant.
    D. Corticosteroid.

12. When selecting a medication to treat dyspnea, which of the following is true?
    A. Antibiotics will relieve feelings of breathlessness.
    B. Antidepressants work within 1 to 2 days.
    C. Benzodiazepines treat the anxiety related to dyspnea.
    D. Corticosteroids will decrease insomnia if given later in the day.

8. **Answer:** There is no definitive answer. Hepatotoxicity in larger doses or with hepatic dysfunction (acetaminophen overdose is the leading cause of acute liver failure in the United States) can also compromise renal function. Formerly the limit on the total amount of acetaminophen that can be given in a 24-hour period was considered to be 4000 mg/day but because this was not based on longitudinal studies, lower doses (3000 mg/day) are recommended for chronic use, including in older/debilitated individuals, alcoholic patients, people with HIV, patients with liver metastasis, or those with active liver disease. Dose escalation is limited by the quantity of acetaminophen in combination medications (e.g., oxycodone/acetaminophen [Percocet], hydromorphone/acetaminophen [Vicodin], over-the-counter cold medications). The U.S. Food and Drug Administration (FDA) warns against having more than 325 mg of acetaminophen per tablet, capsule, or other dosage in medications that contain acetaminophen and another drug.

9. **Answer:**

    - The patches should be placed over intact skin only.
    - Up to 3 patches can be used to cover the painful area; package insert instructs to apply for 12 hours and then remove for 12 hours, but it is safe to leave in place for 18 to 24 hours.
    - Adverse effects are uncommon and include pain with removal of the patch.
    - Patients with sensitivity to touch (also called allodynia) often report relief.

10. **Answer:** Extrapyramidal symptoms (EPS) are involuntary movements, which may not respond to therapies. Along with being uncomfortable, EPS places patients at increased risk for falls, can decrease their ability to do their own activities of daily living (ADLs), and create anxiety. Medications: dopamine D-2 receptor antagonists, first-generation antipsychotics, neuroleptics, butyrophenones (e.g., haloperidol), phenothiazines (e.g., chlorpromazine), prokinetics (e.g., metoclopramide), and opioids.

11. Answer is C

    A. Incorrect: Guaifenesin is not an antibiotic.

    B. Incorrect: Guaifenesin is neither a centrally or peripherally acting antitussive.

    C. **Correct:** Guaifenesin thins secretions to ease expectoration of mucous.

    D. Incorrect: Guaifenesin is not a corticosteroid.

12. Answer is C

    A. Incorrect: Antibiotics may significantly reduce dyspnea caused by an infection.

    B. Incorrect: Antidepressants effects may take weeks to manifest. Treating depression may help with coping but will not improve symptom of dyspnea.

    C. **Correct:** Benzodiazepines do not directly decrease dyspnea but can decrease anxiety, which can make dyspnea worse.

    D. Incorrect: Corticosteroids may disrupt sleep if given late in the day.

13. Methylnaltrexone
    A. Cannot be crushed.
    B. Delays gastrointestinal transit time.
    C. Inhibits opioid induced gastrointestinal slower motility.
    D. Is given orally.

14. When using loperamide to treat diarrhea, the maximum dose per day should not exceed
    A. 6 mg.
    B. 16 mg.
    C. 20 mg.
    D. Administer after each loose stool regardless of amount needed per day.

15. The use of octreotide to treat diarrhea is especially helpful in which of the following conditions?
    A. Bowel obstructions
    B. Conditions that cause increased peristalsis
    C. Late stage human immunodeficiency virus (HIV)
    D. Ulcerative colitis

16. Which of the following should be included when teaching a hospice patient about baclofen for hiccoughs?
    A. "Call the 24-hour hospice phone number if you experience difficulty sleeping, dizziness, difficulty with coordination, or confusion."
    B. "Call the 24-hour hospice phone number if you experience involuntary movements."
    C. "If you have difficulty swallowing the pill, your prescription can be changed to subcutaneous injection."
    D. "We will start you on 300 mg 2 to 3 times per day. If there is no relief from the hiccoughs, call the 24-hour hospice phone number and the doctor can increase the dose."

13. Answer is C

    A. Incorrect: Methylnaltrexone is only given subcutaneously.

    B. Incorrect: Methylnaltrexone inhibits opioid-caused delay in gastrointestinal transit time.

    C. **Correct:** Methylnaltrexone inhibits opioid-induced gastrointestinal slower motility.

    D. Incorrect: Methylnaltrexone is only given subcutaneously.

14. Answer is B

    A. Incorrect: See B.

    B. **Correct:** The correct dosing of loperamide is 4 mg followed by 2 mg after each loose stool, not to exceed 16 mg per day.

    C. Incorrect: The maximum per day dose of diphenoxylate and atropine is 20 mg per day.

    D. Incorrect: See B.

15. Answer is C

    A. Incorrect: Corticosteroids can aid in treating diarrhea by decreasing the inflammation caused by a partial bowel obstruction.

    B. Incorrect: Octreotide does not decrease peristalsis.

    C. **Correct:** Octreotide can aid in treating diarrhea by decreasing gastrointestinal secretions in persons with late stage human immunodeficiency virus (HIV).

    D. Incorrect: Corticosteroids can aid in treating diarrhea by decreasing the inflammation caused by ulcerative colitis.

16. Answer is A

    A. **Correct:** Baclofen can cause sedation, insomnia, ataxia, and mental confusion.

    B. Incorrect: Involuntary movements are more likely a sign of extrapyramidal effects, a side effect of haloperidol.

    C. Incorrect: Baclofen is not available as a subcutaneous injection. Chlorpromazine and haloperidol can be given orally, intravenously, and subcutaneously.

    D. Incorrect: Baclofen doses start at 10 mg 2 to 3 times per day. Gabapentin starts at 300 mg per day in divided doses.

17. Mrs. Gregory has nausea related to gastric stasis. Which class of antiemetics would be recommended?

    A. Antihistamines

    B. Dopamine antagonists

    C. Prokinetic agents

    D. Selective serotonin (5-HT$_3$) receptor antagonists

18. Which of the following is an example of a prokinetic agent?

    A. Cyclizine

    B. Metoclopramide

    C. Ondansetron

    D. Prochlorperazine

19. Which of the following is a starting dose for oral metoclopramide to treat nausea in an adult?

    A. 2 mg every 6 hours

    B. 5 mg every 4 hours

    C. 8 mg twice a day

    D. 10 mg every 8 hours

20. Teaching for a patient using bupropion for fatigue should include the potential for

    A. Abuse.

    B. Gastrointestinal side effects.

    C. Cardiovascular side effects.

    D. Thromboembolic events.

21. Which of the following medications is a first-line agent for delirium?

    A. Haloperidol

    B. Lorazepam

    C. Olanzapine

    D. Risperidone

17. Answer is C

    A. Incorrect: Diphenhydramine is used to treat nausea from intestinal obstruction and increased intracranial pressure. Cyclizine is used to treat nausea from peritoneal irritation and vestibular causes.

    B. Incorrect: Dopamine antagonists block dopamine at the chemoreceptor trigger zone, which can aid in decreasing nausea from chemotherapy and other medications.

    C. **Correct:** Prokinetic agents aid in stimulating motility of the upper gastrointestinal tract.

    D. Incorrect: 5-HT$_3$ receptor antagonists block 5-HT (serotonin) in the central nervous system in the chemotherapy trigger zone and in the peripheral nervous system on nerve terminals of the vagus nerve.

18. Answer is B

    A. Incorrect: Cyclizine is an antihistamine.

    B. **Correct:** Metoclopramide is a prokinetic agent (i.e., stimulates motility of the upper gastrointestinal tract).

    C. Incorrect: Ondansetron is 5-HT$_3$ receptor antagonist.

    D. Incorrect: Prochlorperazine is a dopamine antagonist.

19. Answer is D

    A. Incorrect: 2 mg every 6 hours is a starting dose for dronabinol.

    B. Incorrect: 5 mg every 4 hours is a starting dose for prochlorperazine.

    C. Incorrect: 8 mg twice a day is a starting dose for ondansetron.

    D. **Correct:** 10 mg every 8 hours is a starting dose for metoclopramide.

20. Answer is C

    A. Incorrect: Bupropion does not have an abuse potential. Methylphenidate does.

    B. Incorrect: Bupropion side effects do not include gastrointestinal side effects. Donepezil does.

    C. **Correct:** Bupropion side effects include cardiovascular effects (e.g., hypertension, tachycardia).

    D. Incorrect: Bupropion side effects do not include thromboembolic events. Erythropoietin does.

21. Answer is A

    A. **Correct:** Haloperidol, a neuroleptic, is a first-line medication for delirium.

    B. Incorrect: Lorazepam, a benzodiazepine, has the potential for paradoxical worsening of symptoms, except in cases of suspected alcohol withdrawal.

    C. Incorrect: There is little evidence supporting the use of olanzapine, a new atypical neuroleptic, in treating delirium.

    D. Incorrect: There is little evidence supporting the use of risperidone, a new atypical neuroleptic, in treating delirium.

22. Which of the following correctly describes the action of acetaminophen?

    A. Anticholinergic

    B. Anti-inflammatory

    C. Antipyretic

    D. Inhibits platelet aggregation

23. The black box warning for celecoxib includes

    A. Bronchospasm.

    B. Cardiovascular events.

    C. Renal insufficiency.

    D. Tinnitus.

24. Partial agonist opioids

    A. Have an analgesic ceiling.

    B. Have the same precautions as pure opioids.

    C. May precipitate withdrawal when given to patients who have been on pure mu opioid agonists.

    D. Have psychomimetic actions.

25. Which of the following is the only side effect of opioids that is not time limited?

    A. Constipation

    B. Dysphoria

    C. Nausea

    D. Respiratory depression

22. Answer is C

    A. Incorrect: Acetaminophen does not have anticholinergic effects. Tricyclic antidepressants do.

    B. Incorrect: Acetaminophen does not have any anti-inflammatory properties. Nonsteroidal anti-inflammatory drugs (NSAIDs) and corticosteroids do.

    C. **Correct:** Acetaminophen does have antipyretic properties.

    D. Incorrect: Acetaminophen does not inhibit platelet aggregation. NSAIDs do.

23. Answer is B

    A. Incorrect: Bronchospasm is a potential adverse effect of all nonsteroidal anti-inflammatory drugs (NSAIDs), but is not a black box warning for celecoxib.

    B. **Correct:** The black box warning for celecoxib includes cardiovascular events and gastrointestinal bleeds, though these are potential adverse effects for all NSAIDs.

    C. Incorrect: Renal insufficiency is a potential adverse effect of all NSAIDs, but is not a black box warning for celecoxib.

    D. Incorrect: Tinnitus is a potential adverse effect of all NSAIDs, but is not a black box warning for celecoxib.

24. Answer is B

    A. Incorrect: Mixed agonist-antagonists have an analgesic ceiling, partial agonists do not.

    B. **Correct:** Partial agonists do have the same precautions as pure opioids.

    C. Incorrect: Withdrawal may be precipitated when mixed agonist-antagonists are given to patients who have been on pure mu opioids.

    D. Incorrect: Mixed agonist-antagonists have psychomimetic actions, partial agonists do not.

25. Answer is A

    A. **Correct:** Tolerance does not develop to opioid-induced constipation.

    B. Incorrect: If dysphoria is present upon initiation of an opioid, it will diminish over time.

    C. Incorrect: If nausea is present upon initiation of an opioid, it will diminish over time.

    D. Incorrect: Clinically significant respiratory depression is extremely rare when patients in severe pain receive opioids as ordered. If respiratory depression is present, it may be related to other factors including level of sedation and adequacy of perfusion.

26. Mr. Conti, a new hospice patient, has come to the emergency department due to sedation and respiratory depression related to confusing his short- and long-acting oxycodone. A slow, diluted naloxone infusion has been ordered. What is the expected effect on his pain?

   A. Mr. Conti's pain will remain somewhat controlled.
   B. Pain will return, but can be controlled by switching to another opioid.
   C. Return of all pain until the naloxone wears off in several hours.
   D. The naloxone will create a rapid abstinence syndrome.

27. Which statement is true regarding hydromorphone 3-glucuronide (H3G), an active metabolite of hydromorphone? H3G

   A. Can be cleared by intravenous hydration of 100 to 150 mL/hour.
   B. Has different properties than morphine 3-glucuronide (M3G).
   C. Has no analgesic properties.
   D. Is excreted by the kidneys.

28. Mr. Barber's pain medication has been changed to sublingual morphine as he has been unable to swallow safely. Of the following statements made to his wife, which one indicates that the nurse understands sublingual delivery of morphine?

   A. "Drop the concentrated morphine 1 drop at a time between his cheek and gums."
   B. "Put the concentrated morphine under your husband's tongue so that it can be absorbed."
   C. "I will call the doctor as this is not an appropriate prescription for your husband as he cannot swallow."
   D. "Place the morphine in his mouth and it will trickle down his throat where it will be absorbed in the gastrointestinal tract."

29. Which of the following patients is the best candidate for using a transdermal fentanyl patch?

   A. A 23-year-old man just starting on opioid pain medications.
   B. A 30-year-old in severe pain.
   C. A 48-year-old overweight woman needing frequent opioid dose adjustments.
   D. An 86-year-old man who has been on long-acting opioids for 4 months and whose pain is stable.

26. Answer is A

   A. **Correct:** A bolus of naloxone would completely block binding of all opioids producing abstinence syndrome and return of pain. A slow dilute infusion will allow some pain relief to remain.

   B. Incorrect: Naloxone will affect all opioids.

   C. Incorrect: Had the dose been given via bolus, it would take several hours for the naloxone to wear off before additional pain medication can be given.

   D. Incorrect: A slow dilute infusion will not result in abstinence syndrome.

27. Answer is D

   A. Incorrect: Only a small amount of intervenous hydration (30–50 mL/hour) is needed to clear the metabolite.

   B. Incorrect: Hydromorphone 3-glucuronide (H3G) and morphine 3-glucuronide (M3G) have the same properties.

   C. Incorrect: H3G has strong analgesic properties.

   D. **Correct:** H3G is excreted by the kidneys.

28. Answer is D

   A. Incorrect: The solution is concentrated so that it is of a small enough volume that can be delivered all at once.

   B. Incorrect: Though it can be put under the tongue, most of the concentrated morphine will be absorbed by the gastrointestinal tract.

   C. Incorrect: Sublingual delivery of concentrated opioids is an effective method of route for patients who have difficulty swallowing.

   D. **Correct:** Most of the concentrated morphine will be absorbed by the gastrointestinal tract.

29. Answer is D

   A. Incorrect: Transdermal fentanyl patches should not be used on opioid naïve patients.

   B. Incorrect: Transdermal fentanyl patches have a delayed onset of action of 12 to 24 hours and will not provide pain relief soon enough for someone with severe pain.

   C. Incorrect: Transdermal fentanyl patches should not be used on patients with unstable pain.

   D. **Correct:** Of this list, the best candidate for a transdermal fentanyl patch is someone who has stable pain. Age is not a determining factor.

30. Mrs. Peretti is taking nortriptyline for pain. Which of the following statements made by the nurse is appropriate?

   A. "Don't be discouraged if you don't see improvement right away."

   B. "If your pain has not improved by the day after tomorrow, call me and we can increase the dose."

   C. "Take the nortriptyline in the morning as it can interfere with your ability to fall asleep."

   D. "We can increase your dose every few days up to 150 mg per day if needed."

31. Give example(s), action(s), and teaching point(s) for each of the types of laxatives listed below.

Type	Example(s)	Action(s)	Teaching Point(s)
Bowel stimulants			
Bulk laxative			
Lubricant laxative			
Osmotic laxative			

32. List an example and the action of each class of medication used for anorexia/cachexia and its indication.

Class	Examples	Action
Cannabinoids		
Corticosteroids		
Gastrokinetic agents		
Progestational agents		

30. **Answer is A**

    A. **Correct:** It may take 3 to 7 days before the analgesic effects of nortriptyline are noted.

    B. Incorrect: See A. In addition, dose adjustments should be made every few days not every other day.

    C. Incorrect: Nortriptyline should be taken at bedtime to capitalize on its sedating properties.

    D. Incorrect: The maximum dose for nortriptyline is 75 to 100 mg per day.

31. **Answer:** Example(s), action(s), and teaching point(s) for each type of laxative listed are below.

Type	Example(s)	Action(s)	Teaching Point(s)
Bowel stimulants	• Bisacodyl • Senna	Increase colon motility	• Can cause severe cramping • Can be given rectally
Bulk laxative	• Carboxymethylcellulose • Fiber • Methylcellulose • Psyllium	Provide bulk to increase mass	• Patient must be able to increase fluid intake
Lubricant laxative	Mineral oil	Lubricates stool surface and softens the stool by penetration	• Patient must be able to increase fluid intake • Can be given rectally
Osmotic laxative	• Lactulose • Magnesium citrate • Magnesium hydroxide • Polyethylene glycol • Sorbitol	Nonabsorbable sugars that exert shift in water in both the small and large intestines	• Can cause severe cramping and discomfort

32. **Answer:** Example and action of each class of medication for anorexia/cachexia are listed below.

Class	Examples	Action
Cannabinoids	Dronabinol	Improves appetite and decreases anxiety
Corticosteroids	Dexamethasone	Improves appetite without typically increasing body mass
Gastrokinetic agents	Metoclopramide	Improves appetite and decreases early satiety
Progestational agents	Megestrol	Improves appetite to assist with weight gain

Conversion Worksheet
Formula for Converting to a New Drug or New Route Using Equianalgesic Table (see Appendix A)

Equianalgesic Conversion Process

(See Chapter IV, Pain Management by Judith A. Paice, PhD, RN in the *Core Curriculum for the Hospice and Palliative Registered Nurse* for more information on opioid equianalgesic conversion, cross tolerance, and breakthrough pain.)

Process	Example
Step 1	
Add up the total amount of the current drug given in 24 hours. • Remember to add in both the scheduled and breakthrough or rescue doses. • Calculate separately if more than 1 drug used.	Converting oral hydrocodone to hydromorphone: the patient is taking 2 tablets of acetaminophen in combination with hydrocodone 5 mg every 4 hours (6 doses/day). Because each tablet contains 5 mg of hydrocodone, 2 contain 10 mg. 6 doses × 10 mg = 60 mg/day of hydrocodone
Step 2	
Divide current 24-hour total by the equianalgesic value for the current drug and route of administration (see Appendix A).	60 mg of hydrocodone ÷ 30 mg (equivalent value for hydrocodone) = 2
Step 3	
Multiply the Step 2 number by the equianalgesic value for the new drug and route. • This will give you the new 24-hour dose.	2 × 7.5 mg (equivalent value for oral hydromorphone) = 15 mg (or 15 mg of hydromorphone in 24 hours)
Step 4	
Determine how many doses the patient will take each day and divide this number into the total 24-hour dose. • This gives the amount of medication needed per dose.	Hydromorphone can be given every 4 hours, which is 6 doses a day; divide the 24-hour dose by 6 doses. 15 ÷ 6 = 2.5 2.5 mg hydromorphone every 4 hours; as hydromorphone comes in 2, 4, and 8 mg tablets, round the dose down to 2 mg, have the appropriate breakthrough medications ordered, and carefully monitor the patient for the need to increase the dose.

Alternative Process

$$\frac{\text{Current 24-hour dose}}{\text{Current equivalent \#}} \times \text{New equivalent \#} = \text{New 24-hour dose}$$

Calculating Breakthrough Dose

Oral: 10% to 20% of 24-hour dose available every 1 to 2 hours as needed.

Parenteral: 50% to 100% of the hourly rate every 15 minutes for most medication (check timing of peak effect).

Problem 1

Ms. Gregory has been taking extended release morphine 30 mg every 12 hours for severe pain. She is having myoclonus, most likely from the oral morphine, and an order has been written to switch her to oral oxycodone. What should her controlled-release oxycodone dose be?

Problem 2

Mr. Marcus' pain has been well controlled with a continuous morphine infusion of 5 mg per hour. An order has been written to switch Mr. Marcus to oral morphine. What should his dose of oral morphine be?

Problem 1 Answer

Step 1: Add up the total amount of the current drug given in 24 hours.

30 mg × 2 = 60 mg total in 24 hours

Step 2: Divide the current 24-hour total by the equianalgesic value for the current drug and route of administration.

60 mg of morphine ÷ 30 mg (equivalent value for morphine) = 2

Step 3: Multiply the Step 2 number by the equianalgesic value for the new drug and route, which will give you the new 24-hour dose.

2 × 20 mg (equivalent for oxycodone) = 40 mg of oxycodone per 24 hours

Step 4: Determine how many doses the patient will take each day and divide this number into the total 24-hour dose, which gives the amount of medication needed per dose.
Controlled-release oxycodone can be given every 12 hours, which is 2 doses per day; divide the 24-hour dose by 2.

40 mg ÷ 2 = 20 mg per dose

Problem 2 Answer

5 mg/hour × 24 hours = 120 mg/day

120 mg of morphine ÷ 10 mg (equivalent for parenteral morphine) = 12

12 × 30 mg (equivalent for oral morphine) = 360 mg

360 mg ÷ 6 doses per day = 60 mg/dose or 2 30 mg morphine tablets every 4 hours

If a long-acting morphine is desired, his dose would be 180 mg orally every 12 hours.

Problem 3

Though Ms. Martin's pain had been well controlled on 5 mg hydrocodone/300 mg acetaminophen 2 tablets every 6 hours, she is now having difficulty swallowing and is being switched to liquid oxycodone. What should her dose of oxycodone be?

Problem 4

Mrs. Peters, a 58-year-old woman on hospice with a diagnosis of metastatic breast cancer, is taking oral hydromorphone extended-release 3 16 mg tablets daily. She developed mouth sores and is to be switched to intravenous (IV) hydromorphone. What will her per hourly IV rate be?

Problem 5

Mrs. Soter is a 93-year-old woman new to hospice with a diagnosis of thyroid cancer. Upon admission, her pain was well controlled on 10 mg morphine oral solution 8 times per day. Admission orders include switching her to morphine extended-release pellets twice a day so she can sleep through the night. What would her dose of extended-release morphine be?

What should be ordered for the lowest breakthrough dose?

Problem 3 Answer

5 mg of hydrocodone per tablet = 10 mg hydrocodone per dose

10 mg hydrocodone per dose × 4 doses per day = 40 mg of hydrocodone per 24 hours

40 mg ÷ 30 mg = 1.3

1.3 × 20 = 26 mg/24 hours

Because Ms. Martin's pain is well controlled, the dose of the new drug will be decreased by 25% to account for incomplete cross tolerance

26 × 0.25 = 6.5

26 − 6.5 = 19.5 mg/day

Oxycodone oral solution is available in 5 mg/5 mL and 20 mg/mL. Because Ms. Martin is having difficulty swallowing, the higher concentrated solution will be used.

20 mg/mL

19.5 mg/day is close enough to 20 mg/day

20 mg ÷ 4 doses/day = 5 mg/dose

5 mg/dose of 20 mg/mL = 0.25 mL every 6 hours

Problem 4 Answer

3 × 16 = 48

48 ÷ 7.5 = 6.4

6.4 × 1.5 = 9.6

9.6 ÷ 24 = 0.4 mg/hour

Problem 5 Answer

10 × 8 = 24-hour dose of liquid morphine is 80 mg

80 mg ÷ 2 = 40 mg every 12 hours of extended-release morphine

Breakthrough dose

80 mg × 10% = 8 mg every 2 hours

Problem 6

Mr. Lyon's pain has been challenging to manage. After trying multiple oral medications, the team has determined that an IV infusion of morphine would be necessary to control his pain. He is currently taking hydromorphone 64 mg once per day with 8 mg hydromorphone 6 times a day for breakthrough pain. What should his IV morphine dose be?

What should the breakthrough dose be?

Problem 7

Mrs. Nicholas' pain had been controlled on extended-release morphine 30 mg twice a day by mouth. She has developed a partial bowel obstruction and needs to be switched to concentrated liquid morphine. What should her new morphine dosage be?

Problem 6 Answer

64 mg + 48 mg = 112 mg/24 hours

112 ÷ 7.5 mg = 15

15 × 10 = 150

150 mg/24 hours IV = 6 mg/hour

Breakthrough dose

As Mr. Lyons is just starting on IV pain medication, 50% of the hourly rate will be used for breakthrough pain.

6 mg × 0.5 = 3 mg every 15 minutes

Problem 7 Answer

30 mg × 2 doses = 60 mg/day of morphine

60 ÷ 4 = 15 mg every 6 hours

Concentrated liquid morphine is available in 20 mg/mL and 100 mg/5 mL

Using either concentration, the dose would be 0.75 mL

Problem 8

Ms. Victor is a 36-year-old woman with hepatoma and end stage liver disease. She has a history of illicit drug abuse including PCP, which she used as recently as 2 weeks ago. Today the patient rates her pain at a 6 on a scale of 1 to 10. She has been discharged home on MS Contin 30 mg orally every 12 hours with immediate release morphine 30 mg tablets every 2 hours for breakthrough pain. After reading her admission history and physical and other information, you find out that on the day of discharge from the hospital she was receiving 8 mg IV morphine every hour for pain. You also determine that she has been taking as much as 60 mg MS Contin every 8 hours routinely for pain. The patient has good renal function and is slender. What information is missing?

Assessment determines she denies further PCP use, her pain was controlled in the hospital, she has been taking the breakthrough doses 5 times per day, and she states her pain is now controlled. The team is concerned she is abusing the morphine. Do you concur?

What are your recommendations for her pain regimen?

Problem 8 Answer

Missing information: How many times per day is she taking the breakthrough pain medication, complete assessment of her current pain, is she using PCP or other street drugs currently, was her pain controlled on her hospital dose?

To determine if she is abusing the morphine, her hospital, ordered, and actual 24-hour totals of morphine need to be calculated.

Hospital 24-hour total:

   8 mg × 24 = 192 mg/24 hours of IV morphine

   192 ÷ 10 = 19.2

   19.2 × 30 = 576 mg/24 hours oral morphine equivalent

Ordered oral morphine total if taking maximum amount of breakthrough dosing:

   60 + 360 = 420 mg/24 hours oral

Actual morphine total:

   180 + 150 = 330 mg/24 hours oral

Conclusion: In the hospital, Ms. Victor was taking the oral equivalent of 576 mg morphine per day, but was discharged on only 180 mg morphine/day plus breakthrough dosing. Her actual morphine oral total is 330 mg, which is below what she had been taking in the hospital, and is effective for controlling her pain.

Recommendations: Though what she is currently taking is working, the MS Contin should only be taken twice a day and the amount of breakthrough pain doses indicates that her scheduled dose should be increased. This could be accomplished by increasing the morphine and allay fears of misuse by using 2 80 mg morphine/3.2 mg naltrexone capsules every 12 hours with 30 mg immediate-release for breakthrough pain.

Appendix A
Opioid Dosing
Equivalence

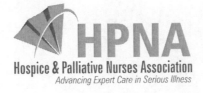

Approximate Equianalgesic Doses of Most Commonly Used Opioid Analgesics[adapted from 1]

Drug	Parenteral Route	Enteral Route
Morphine[†]	10 mg	30 mg
Codeine	130 mg	200 mg (not recommended)
Fentanyl[‡††]	50–100 mcg	TIRF[‡]
Hydrocodone	Not available	30 mg
Hydromorphone[§]	1.5 mg	7.5 mg
Levorphanol[¶]	2 mg acute, 1 chronic	4 mg acute, 1 chronic
Methadone[¶*]	Unknown	Unknown
Oxycodone[**]	Not available	20 mg

[†]Available in continuous and sustained-release pills and capsules, formulated to last 12 or 24 hours.

[‡]Also available in transdermal and transmucosal immediate release fentanyl (TIRF), see package insert materials for dose recommendations.

[††]Fentanyl 100 mcg patch ≈ 2–3 mg intravenous morphine/hour.[2]

[§]Available as a continuous-release formulation lasting 24 hours.

[¶]These drugs have long half-lives, so accumulation can occur; close monitoring during first few days of therapy is very important.

[*]Because equipotent ratios for methadone are unknown, many recommend starting the oral dose at 2.5–5 mg every 8 hours (1/2 dose for elderly or severe renal or liver disease: 1.25–2.5 mg)[3] regardless of the previous opioid dose; do not titrate any more frequently than every 3–7 days; provide sufficient immediate release opioids for breakthrough pain. Methadone can prolong the QT interval. The general guideline is to avoid methadone if QT is approaching or exceeding 500. The frequency of electrocardiography (ECG) monitoring depends on the patient's goals of care.

[**]Available in several continuous-release doses, formulated to last 12 hours.

CITED REFERENCES

1. Paice JA. Pain at the end of life. In: Ferrell B, Coyle N, Paice JA, eds. *Oxford Textbook of Palliative Nursing*. 4th ed. New York, NY: Oxford University Press. 2015:in press.

2. McPherson ML. *Demystifying Opioid Conversion Calculations: A Guide for Effective Dosing*. Bethesda, MD: American Society of Health-System Pharmacists; 2010.

3. Quill TE, Holloway RG, Shah MS, Caprio TV, Olden AM, Storey CP. *Primer of Palliative Care*. 5th ed. Glenview, IL: American Academy of Hospice and Palliative Medicine; 2010.

Appendix B

Test Taking and Study Skills—Preparation for Success

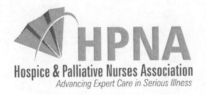

Test Taking and Study Skills—Preparation for Success

Important Reading and Viewing

- *Certified Hospice and Palliative Nurse (CHPN®) Candidate Handbook*—instructions for applying for the exam; fees; detailed content outline; study advice; what to do on the day of the exam; sample questions; suggested references; and much more (hpcc.advancingexpertcare.org/competence/rn-chpn/)

- *Applied Measurement Professionals, Inc. (AMP)*—*What to Expect* video and *General Recommendations* from the testing agency (goamp.com/Pages/Candidate-Information.aspx)

- *Secrets of Competency Testing: Writing Items for Hospice and Palliative Certification Exams—Session 1 and Session 2*—by learning how to write exam questions, test takers may feel more confident on exam day (nurseslearning.com/catalog.cfm?Topic=40%20)

I. Understand yourself

    A. Recall past experiences with studying for and taking a big exam. Do you procrastinate studying? Do you become anxious and have difficulty concentrating? Are you overconfident? Do exam situations pose no threat to you?

    B. Reflect on *your* years of experience

    C. Use the CHPN® detailed content outline (hpcc.advancingexpertcare.org/competence/rn-chpn/) to do a self-assessment of your knowledge. Base your study plan on the results of your self-assessment; start with the weaker areas first as people have a tendency to study what they already know

        1. All questions are based on an item from the detailed content outline

        2. Be aware of the weight of content areas. For example, 24% of the questions will be on *Patient Care: Pain Management*, while 7% are on *Professional Issues*

    D. Do not listen to gossip about the exam—keep your focus

        1. Doing an Internet search for help in passing exams may give you a lot of study tips, but do not let this keep you from studying. Use only reputable sites (e.g., universities, professional organizations)

    E. Study with others if that is how you learn best

II. Develop your memory/recall skills. These are more powerful and effective if you can think of your own!

    A. Acronyms example—each letter of a word is the first letter of a related word (e.g., DYSPNEA can be exacerbated by Depression; Yearning for peace, rest, and forgiveness; Social issues; Physical problems; Nonacceptance or spiritual distress; Economic or financial distress; Anxiety/Anger)

B. Acrostics—catchy phrases where the first letter of each word stands for what is to be recalled (e.g., the phrase for remembering the cranial nerves—"On old Olympus towering tops a Fin and German viewed some hops," where each word's first letter is the first letter of the cranial nerve)

C. Imaging—think of a nickname for a disease, situation, or a specific patient you have cared for with that disease or situation

D. Rhymes, music, and links—linking content with fun jingles, songs, or through a story can be helpful in learning and remembering

E. Use of color highlighters or drawing can improve recall; making colors meaningful can also help (blue for respiratory, red for regulatory [i.e., "red tape"])

III. Build a study plan based on your strengths and weaknesses

A. Create a study schedule
1. Develop a timeline for studying (e.g., what you will do 6 months before the exam, 3 months before, 1 month before). Allocate time to review each of the examination content areas. Stick to the study plan
2. Plan the study time that suits your needs. If you are a morning person, study in the morning hours. Study in short "bursts" alternating with stretching or taking a walk
3. The study area should be quiet, without distractions, and include a few breaks in the schedule
4. Avoid the "forgetting curve"—without use or review, retention of learned material decreases[1]
   a. Find ways to "use" the information as you learn it (e.g., think of previous or current patients that would benefit from what you just learned)

B. Study methods—find 1 or more that work best for you, but do not spread yourself to thin[2]
1. Individual study using the many available resources; take notes; highlight a textbook; prepare quiz cards; audio record you reading a resource and listen to the tapes
2. Studying with a partner or in a group—along with the available resources, consider challenging each other by writing your own test questions and case studies
3. The Hospice and Palliative Registered Nurse Self-Assessment Examination (RN SAE)—a 50-question online practice examination developed to acquaint potential CHPN® candidates with test taking and allow them to become familiar with the format of the examination (store.lxr.com/product.aspx?id=1238)
4. CHPN® Certification Review Course—a 1-day course encompasses the fundamental concepts of palliative nursing (hpna.advancingexpertcare.org/education/chpn-certification-review-course/)
5. Publications—many books on a variety of palliative care topics (www.hpna.org/HPNA_Shop.aspx)

6. E-learning—over 50 courses on a variety of palliative care topics (hpna.advancingexpertcare.org/education/e-learning/) or free in HPNA Members Only (advancingexpertcare.org/login/)

7. *Journal of Hospice and Palliative Nursing*—current and archived issues available in HPNA Members Only (advancingexpertcare.org/login/)

8. *Journal of Palliative Medicine*—current and archived issues available in HPNA Members Only (advancingexpertcare.org/login/)

9. Position Statements—over 20 topics available (hpna.advancingexpertcare.org/education/position-statements/)

C. Anxiety

1. There are two components of test anxiety—worry (concern about performance) and emotionality (physiological arousal). Do not let yourself become preoccupied with either. Keep your focus on preparation[3]

2. On the day of the examination, a brief review of the material may be helpful but a long study session can be counterproductive

3. Prepare a checklist of items needed to take to the test (e.g., photo identification, registration slip). Review the *Candidate Handbook* for details

4. Do not bring many items into the testing center. You can only take your wallet and keys with you into the testing area

5. Be familiar with the location, traffic patterns, and parking facilities of the testing site (in advance of the testing day)

6. Plan to arrive at the test site early in case of unexpected delays. If you are more than 15 minutes late, you will not be able to take the exam and will forfeit your fee

IV. Multiple choice test questions

A. All questions on the CHPN® exam are multiple choice

B. Multiple choice questions have 3 parts: background statement, stem, and options for the answer

1. Background statement—provides information that will assist in answering the question

2. Stem—asks (or states the intent of) the question

3. Options for answer—4 options; 1 is correct and the others serve as "distracters"

C. Tips

1. Identify the purpose of the test question—most questions intend either to measure memory/recall (knowledge of facts) or comprehension/application (ability to use information)

2. Read the stem very carefully—it contains all the information you need to answer the question. Do not add information just because you think it should be there

3. Read every option/answer carefully

4. Resist second guessing—bookmark questions for further thought, sometimes you can find the answer to the question in subsequent questions

5. When you do not know the right answer, eliminate the wrong ones, often you can narrow the choices down to 2—and increase your odds of guessing the right answer

6. Do not eliminate an answer unless you know what all words mean

7. If you do not know the answer—guess—an unanswered question is automatically wrong, there is no penalty for guessing

8. Manage your time carefully—watches cannot be worn in the testing area but you can check your time remaining on the screen

9. You can make comments on items that you have questions about, but do not let this take up too much of your testing time

10. More can be found at *Secrets of Competency Testing: Writing Items for Hospice and Palliative Certification Exams—Session 1 and Session 2*—by learning how to write exam questions, test takers may feel more confident on exam day (nurseslearning.com/catalog.cfm?Topic=40%20)

11. Push yourself on—do not allow yourself to become stymied by 1 question

12. Try these 2 examples—answers can be found just before the references

Examples:

1. Which international political figure has ties to Utah?

    A. Desmond Tutu

    B. Diane Sawyer

    C. Orrin Hatch

    D. The Dalai Lama

2. A patient begins to experience a severe gastrointestinal hemorrhage. The priority intervention in the plan of care to meet the patient's fluid needs should include which of the following?

    A. Accommodating the patient's frequent need for the bedpan or emesis basin

    B. Maintaining gastric pH

    C. Rapidly administering blood and fluid

    D. Monitoring the vital signs on an hourly basis

V. Words of encouragement and tips for success

   A. Remember the exam measures *minimally* competent, not expert, practice

   B. Always be mindful the exam tests the *national* standard of practice, not local customs or practices—they can vary widely

- C. Disease progression is more important to know than disease pathology

- D. Have a working knowledge of the more unusual diagnoses or the ones that you are not familiar with

- E. Study generic names of medications

- F. Agree to support one another no matter who passes or fails

- G. When you pass, celebrate! Your program may want to issue a press release. Frame and display your certificate. Update your nametag and business cards

- H. If you do not pass, take the exam the very next time. Your chances of passing are higher

VI. Answers to sample questions

Examples:

1. Which international political figure has ties to Utah?
   - A. Desmond Tutu
   - B. Diane Sawyer
   - C. Orrin Hatch
   - D. The Dalai Lama

   Answer D—even if you do not have any idea what the right answer is, "international political figure" is the key here, which narrows it down to A & D; if you still do not know then guess.

2. A patient begins to experience a severe gastrointestinal hemorrhage. The priority intervention in the plan of care to meet the patient's fluid needs should include which of the following?
   - A. Accommodating the patient's frequent need for the bedpan or emesis basin
   - B. Maintaining gastric pH
   - C. Rapidly administering blood and fluid
   - D. Monitoring the vital signs on an hourly basis

   Answer C—"as a priority" is the key here; go with your basic nursing knowledge. You can rule out the ones that are wrong and go from there

CITED REFERENCES

1. Custers EJ, Ten Cate OT. Very long-term retention of basic science knowledge in doctors after graduation. *Med Educ*. 2011;45(4):422-430. doi: 10.1111/j.1365-2923.2010.03889.x.

2. Encandela J, Gibson C, Angoff N, Leydon G, Green M. Characteristics of test anxiety among medical students and congruence of strategies to address it. *Med Educ Online*. 2014;19:25211. doi: 10.3402/meo.v19.25211.

3. Damer DE, Melendres LT. "Tackling Test Anxiety": a group for college students. *J Specialists Group Work*. 2011;36(3):163-177. doi: 10.1080/01933922.2011.586016.

Appendix C

Practice Exam

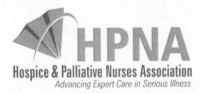

Practice Exam Questions

Directions—Find uninterrupted time to work through all the questions, then grade yourself using the answers that follow the last question. *This section is for practicing your exam taking skills and is not intended to predict exam results.*

Note—Each question is representative of a domain of the CHPN® Detailed Content Outline, which is indicated by the numbers and letter in parentheses in the first line of the answer. For example, (3A2) refers to 3. Patient Care: Symptom Management; A. Neurological; 2. dysphagia. The complete content outline can be found at hpna.advancingexpertcare.org/wp-content/uploads/2014/12/HPCC-CHPN-Handbook-January-2015_CM4.pdf.

1. The family of a 72-year-old woman calls the on-call hospice nurse at 3 AM because they believe her decline is due to her recently increased dose of morphine. Which assessment findings would most strongly suggest an issue with the morphine?

    A. Decreased level of consciousness

    B. Myoclonus

    C. Hyperventilation

    D. Periodic apnea and diaphoresis

2. Which cancer is the LEAST likely to metastasize to the bone?

    A. Lung

    B. Colorectal

    C. Prostate

    D. Breast

3. The drug of choice to relieve the patient's feeling of "air hunger" in end stage pulmonary disease is

    A. Meperidine.

    B. Lorazepam.

    C. Albuterol.

    D. Morphine.

4. A 63-year-old woman receiving hospice care has advanced lung cancer and is experiencing new dyspnea. She has a past medical history of heart failure and has been taking digoxin and furosemide. Which of the following is the first step in addressing her dyspnea?

    A. Call the physician to request an order for morphine.

    B. Hold all medications, position patient in semi/high Fowler's, and reassess in 24 hours.

    C. Inquire if the patient has been taking her medications for heart failure.

    D. Reassure the patient and family that this is part of the normal disease progression.

5. A 54-year-old woman has end stage ovarian cancer. During the hospice nurse's home visit today, she reports a 3-day history of vomiting. She has an increased abdominal girth and reports abdominal discomfort. She also has had no bowel movement in days. Which is most likely to be occurring?

   A. Medication side effects

   B. Bowel obstruction

   C. Spinal cord compression

   D. Pleural effusion

6. Which of the following is NOT an appropriate intervention for a bowel obstruction?

   A. Nasogastric tube to suction

   B. Corticosteroids

   C. Metoclopramide

   D. Octreotide

7. A 90-year-old man is newly admitted to the hospice program in a long-term care facility. He no longer recognizes his family, is bed bound, and presents with extreme rigidity of all extremities. He has developed hypoactive delirium. As the plan of care is initiated, which of the following is an appropriate intervention?

   A. Create an atmosphere with limited stimulation.

   B. Teach and/or reinforce with facility staff the importance of frequent passive range of motion.

   C. Frequent and gentle stimulation (e.g., touch, music).

   D. Discourage family to remain/become involved with care until he settles in.

8. An 86-year-old inpatient hospice patient claims to see his deceased wife and mother, and hears them asking him to "come home." The family is upset and has asked the nurse to sedate him. Which of the following is an appropriate response?

   A. Contact the physician and ask for an order for haloperidol.

   B. Restrain the patient.

   C. Call the chaplain to address the spiritual pain.

   D. Assure the family that "seeing" people who have died is common.

9. The hospice nurse is called to the home of a patient with lung cancer who has the following signs and symptoms: facial edema, dyspnea, and edematous arms with a bluish color. What is most likely happening with this patient?

   A. Allergic reaction to morphine

   B. Superior vena cava syndrome

   C. Congestive heart failure

   D. Pneumonia

10. The process of psychological, social, and somatic reactions to a perceived future loss is known as

    A. Mourning.
    B. Grief.
    C. Bereavement.
    D. Anticipatory grief.

11. Which of following is the best indication of pain relief for a resident with dementia in a nursing home?

    A. Resumes her usual wandering in the hallway
    B. Reports by nursing assistants
    C. Decrease in blood pressure
    D. A lower number on a pain scale

12. Signs and symptoms of imminent death include which of the following?

    A. Unable to sleep
    B. Heightened senses
    C. High blood pressure with a weak and irregular pulse
    D. Dysphagia

13. A 53-year-old Asian-American woman is new to a hospice program. She has a diagnosis of metastatic breast cancer. She reports severe pain (9 on a 10-point scale) in her back and right upper abdominal area. The first priority is to

    A. Start liquid morphine.
    B. Start sustained release morphine.
    C. Assess the pain and obtain a history.
    D. Call the doctor.

14. When are nonpharmacological interventions appropriate to use for pain control?

    A. In place of opioids, when the patient is fearful of addiction.
    B. To augment optimal pharmacological management.
    C. To keep the family busy so they will not worry about the patient.
    D. To manage increased pain until the physician is back in the office.

15. A patient has an area of skin on her left heal that is blistered and cracked. What stage of skin breakdown does she have?

    A.   Stage I

    B.   Stage II

    C.   Stage III

    D.   Stage IV

16. The state of having suffered a loss is

    A.   Mourning.

    B.   Grief.

    C.   Bereavement.

    D.   Anticipatory grief.

17. Disseminated intravascular coagulation

    A.   Is a metabolic response to tumor cells being killed rapidly.

    B.   Signs and symptoms include focal ischemia, widespread thrombosis or bleeding, superficial gangrene, and jaundice.

    C.   Treatments include radiation and/or chemotherapy.

    D.   Most commonly occurs in patients with sarcomas, teratomas, mesotheliomas, breast or lung cancer, or hematological malignancies.

18. A 68-year-old man with a prognosis of days to weeks has developed dysphagia. Which of the following is most appropriate in his treatment plan?

    A.   Liquid diet

    B.   Teach his family the importance of oral hygiene

    C.   Video fluoroscopy swallowing study

    D.   Keep mouth moistened with lemon and glycerin swabs

19. When considering the interdisciplinary approach to symptoms, which of the following is true?

    A.   Symptom management must be the first priority of the team.

    B.   The team should address all problems at the same time.

    C.   Spiritual pain always presents as physical pain.

    D.   The nurse is the most important member of the interdisciplinary team.

20. For the patient who has advanced dementia, a priority therapeutic intervention is

    A. Keep TV on to distract the patient from wandering.

    B. Explain every procedure in detail.

    C. Anticipate safety needs.

    D. Encourage frequent naps.

21. A hospice nurse visits a 70-year-old man with heart failure and head and neck cancer for which he was treated with radiation a year ago. He is taking multiple medications, including diuretics, anticholinergics, and antihistamines. These could cause

    A. Xerostomia.

    B. Stomatitis.

    C. Dysphagia.

    D. Esophagitis.

22. A 38-year-old unmarried man has been hospitalized with a seizure due to an aggressive brain tumor diagnosed a year ago. He is intermittently confused and is determined to not be decisional now. He completed an advance directive 6 months ago stating he wishes to have no extraordinary measures. His sister, his next-of-kin, disagrees and requests that "everything possible" be done to prolong his life. The patient's wishes should be

    A. Ignored because the family member disagrees.

    B. Respected as written in the advance directive.

    C. Discussed with family members and respected.

    D. Ignored and aggressive care should be immediately started.

23. Spiritual care of the hospice patient and family

    A. Is provided in accordance with the religion of the hospice chaplain.

    B. Is only provided by a hospice staff member.

    C. Is provided to every patient and family admitted to hospice care.

    D. Identifies and strives to relieve the spiritual suffering of the patient and family.

24. Grief is

    A. A normal reaction to loss.

    B. An overt expression of the loss.

    C. Defined differently among ethnic groups.

    D. Detrimental to dealing with a loss.

25. An example of advocacy in palliative care includes all of the following **EXCEPT**

    A. Testifying about the importance of quality end-of-life care.

    B. Negotiating continuous care reimbursement with a private insurance company.

    C. Disagreeing with team members regarding the need for a change in the level of care.

    D. Assuring a patient that the goals of care that her son wants are most important.

26. Mentoring is

    A. A relationship between an experienced person and a less experienced person.

    B. A passive method of supporting clinicians with less experience.

    C. Direct supervision provided to the clinician.

    D. A collegial, systematic, and periodic process by which clinicians are held accountable for practice.

27. Supervision of nursing assistants includes all of following **EXCEPT**

    A. Review of the care plan.

    B. Observation of care being given.

    C. Documentation of the supervisory visit.

    D. Telling a nursing assistant to not feel burdened.

28. A male 76-year-old patient was admitted to hospice 4 weeks ago. He was diagnosed with colon cancer 4 years ago and elected hospice for relief of his abdominal pain and loss of appetite. In the past week, he has become more fatigued, spends more time in bed, and is unable to bathe or feed himself. His wife is also very tired because she is doing more of the physical care for her husband. What changes should the hospice nurse initiate in the plan of care that would improve quality of life for both patient and wife?

    A. Suggesting a hospice aide visit 3 times a week to help the patient with bathing.

    B. Counsel his wife on her need to rest.

    C. Teach his wife how to give a bed bath.

    D. Decrease his pain medication.

29. Changes in the status of an 82-year-old man on hospice indicate progression of his disease with a prognosis of days to weeks. How would the interdisciplinary team be used to provide coordinated care?

    A. Initiate a referral to the hospice physical therapist for strengthening exercises.

    B. Ask the couple separately if either would like a visit from the social worker.

    C. Arrange for the chaplain to visit.

    D. Encourage his wife to make an appointment for her husband with his attending physician.

30. A 58-year-old man with end stage lung cancer has intact skin but is cachectic and in bed most of the time. His family has requested a very expensive specialty bed when a less expensive option would be as effective. What ethical principle would be used to determine if the very expensive bed should be provided?

    A. Confidentiality

    B. Autonomy

    C. Beneficence

    D. Justice

31. What are the Medicare Hospice Benefit periods?

    A. 30-, 90-, and 90-day periods

    B. 90-, 90-, and unlimited 90-day periods

    C. 90-, 90-, and unlimited 60-day periods

    D. 30-, 60-, and 90-day periods

32. Which of the following is the best example of crossing of professional boundaries?

    A. Making cookies for a patient.

    B. Providing a personal cell phone number to the family.

    C. Staying an extra half hour to talk to the wife, who is upset.

    D. Praying with a patient who has requested it.

33. A hospice program is very short on nursing staff and the supervisor has requested a hospice nurse work on her day off. The nurse is very fatigued from taking several nights on call but feels committed to the program. What would be her best response in order to meet the needs of the program and take care of herself?

    A. Suggest the supervisor take care of the patients.

    B. Let the supervisor know that she is exhausted and needs the day off.

    C. Do the extra day without saying anything.

    D. Throw her hands up in the air and storm out of the room without answering.

34. A 56-year-old woman on hospice presents to the emergency department for syncope and a recent fall. Which of the following should be considered?

    A. Consider discontinuing antihypertensive medications if blood pressure is consistently low.

    B. Encourage her to remain in bed.

    C. Encourage her to drink less fluid to avoid needing to go to the bathroom.

    D. Restrain her in bed so she cannot fall.

35. An appropriate criterion for deciding to institute any given therapy for a terminally ill patient is if

    A. It is consistent with the patient's goals.

    B. The physician wants to try one more treatment.

    C. The family demands it.

    D. It will prolong life.

36. If the patient decides to revoke the Medicare Hospice Benefit, the patient and family need to know that

    A. Their Medicare Hospice election remains valid if they choose to come back later.

    B. They will lose the remaining days of the current benefit period.

    C. Either the patient (or patient's representative) or the hospice program may revoke the Medicare Hospice Benefit.

    D. Once they revoke the Medicare Hospice Benefit, they are ineligible for it in the future.

37. The dose-limiting side effect of morphine is

    A. Respiratory depression.

    B. Myoclonus.

    C. Constipation.

    D. Dehydration.

38. A 78-year-old has been admitted to the intensive care unit post motor vehicle accident with head trauma, internal bleeding, and is intermittently confused. His wife died as a result of the accident. His next-of-kin is an adult daughter. What is the first step in developing a plan of care?

    A. Did he have prior symptoms of dementia?

    B. What is his decision-making capacity?

    C. Did he have an advance directive?

    D. What are the daughter's wishes for his care?

39. A 21-year-old Cambodian man suffered an anoxic event 5 years ago and has been in a chronic vegetative state since the injury and cared for at home by his very devoted family. He has been admitted to the hospital for the fourth time within the past year for pneumonia. The family is now questioning his quality of life and the palliative care team has been consulted. Of the questions below, which is the first priority to ask the family about their culture? What

    A. Role does healthcare take in healing?

    B. Is the role of the family in making healthcare decisions?

    C. Do Cambodians believe about withdrawing treatment?

    D. Traditional therapies have they been using?

40. What is the appropriate wound care for a stage II pressure ulcer?

    A. Surgical repair

    B. Irrigation and debridement

    C. Apply protective/occlusive dressing

    D. A & D ointment

41. A patient is being switched from oral morphine to oral oxycodone. The patient is on morphine 100 mg every 8 hours and 10 mg for breakthrough pain, which he has used 6 times in the last 24 hours. What will the patient's every 4 hour dose of oxycodone be?

    A. 40 mg

    B. 50 mg

    C. 60 mg

    D. 90 mg

42. The usual cause of death for patients with amyotrophic lateral sclerosis (ALS) is

    A. Lack of nutrition.

    B. Overwhelming infection.

    C. Respiratory failure.

    D. Cholinergic crisis.

43. Patients with chronic renal failure

    A. Are likely to have completed an advance directive.

    B. Are not eligible for hospice until dialysis is discontinued.

    C. Can have their pain managed with morphine.

    D. Maintain cognitive functioning.

44. Which of the following is the most appropriate patient to use a tricyclic antidepressant as an adjuvant analgesic? A patient with

    A. Diarrhea.

    B. Incontinence.

    C. Myoclonus.

    D. Seizures.

45. Which of the following is a barrier to patient communication?

   A. Anticipate what patients will say.

   B. Do not change the topic when the patient becomes upset.

   C. Make sure you address all the points you planned to tell the patient.

   D. Sit quietly during periods of silence.

46. Which of the following statements if made by a family member about her husband would indicate a need for immediate further assessment?

   A. "I know he doesn't sound very hopeful that the pain medication will work but he has always been a 'glass half empty' person."

   B. "He didn't mean what he said about wishing he could end this all now."

   C. "He gets quiet when he needs to think about something. They talked to him about discontinuing his dialysis today."

   D. "I'm sorry he yelled at you. He doesn't like how weak he has been since the stroke."

47. A 94-year-old widow is a resident of a nursing home and newly elected hospice care. She is from a culture that is known for letting the men make healthcare decisions. When planning for the first team meeting, the nurse should

   A. Invite only her eldest son.

   B. Invite only the patient.

   C. Not tell her about the team meeting.

   D. Ask who she wants to attend the team meetings.

48. Which statement made by a nurse indicates that she understands the purpose of a life review? "I see that you are smiling while you listen to the big band music.

   A. Did you ever go to see one of famous big bands?"

   B. Does it have a special meaning for you?"

   C. Does it remind you of your time in the Navy?"

   D. Was big band music played at your wedding?"

49. All of the following are components of burnout **EXCEPT**

   A. Compassion fatigue.

   B. Cynicism and depersonalization.

   C. Emotional exhaustion.

   D. Ineffectiveness and lack of personal accomplishment.

50. A patient has been on intravenous morphine, 2.5 mg/hour. She is now able to take oral medications and will be switched to oral morphine. What will her every 4 hour dose be?

    A. 15 mg

    B. 30 mg

    C. 45 mg

    D. 125 mg

51. Long-term cardiac toxicity of chemotherapy has symptoms similar to

    A. Cardiac tamponade.

    B. Congestive heart failure.

    C. Pleurisy.

    D. Postural hypotension.

52. An assisted living resident with long-standing metastatic prostate cancer to the mid-thoracic vertebrae in the middle of a poker game he is enjoying requests a dose of breakthrough medication. The nurse looks at the medication record and sees he can have a dose of breakthrough pain medication now. The nurse's best action would be to

    A. Be suspicious and consider that he is drug seeking as he knows what "breakthrough pain medication" means.

    B. Recognize that the resident is not in pain as he is enjoying the poker game.

    C. Suggest that resident lay down for a while.

    D. Administer a dose of breakthrough pain medication.

53. A patient with type 1 diabetes and advanced renal failure is considering stopping finger-stick glucose monitoring. Her diabetes is stable on insulin. She asks the nurse for reasons that she might want to continue monitoring her glucose. The nurse responds by

    A. Agreeing that testing is no longer needed.

    B. Suggesting that she continue monitoring as her insulin will need to be increased.

    C. Suggesting that she continue monitoring as hyperglycemia and/or hypoglycemia can affect quality of life.

    D. Telling her that monthly Hb A_1C levels will be adequate to monitor her glucose.

54. Which of the following is a type of pain that is experienced by patients with multiple sclerosis?

    A. Hyperalgesia

    B. Pain associated with deconditioning

    C. Spasmodic pain

    D. Visceral pain

55. In a lecture a nurse learned that Veterans are often stoic and do not report pain. The next day she cares for a Desert Storm Veteran who is not expected to survive severe burns he sustained in a motor vehicle accident. The nurse knows that he must be in pain but he says that he does not have any pain and wants to be left alone. Of the following, which is the nurse's best approach to his pain management?

    A. Ask him if he had bad experiences related to burns during his time in the military.

    B. Give him intravenous pain medication without telling him.

    C. Have the chaplain visit with him.

    D. Normalize the experience of pain and that severe pain is almost universal with burns and discuss the analgesics ordered for him.

56. Brachytherapy is

    A. Low dose chemotherapy.

    B. Implanted radiation therapy.

    C. Medications to raise the blood pressure.

    D. Medications to raise the pulse.

57. What is the 24-hour ceiling dose of acetaminophen for an 80-year-old woman who does not have liver disease?

    A. 325 mg

    B. 1000 mg

    C. 3000 gm

    D. 4000 gm

58. What type of pain typically requires antiepileptics and antidepressants for pain relief?

    A. Visceral

    B. Somatic

    C. Neuropathic

    D. Referred

59. Which statement would be a cause of concern for possible opioid diversion in the household?

    A. "These pills really help my pain. My pain level stays at 2–3 as long as I take my pills like they have been prescribed."

    B. "I take 4 pills each day. Since I have 8 pills left, I need to have my prescription filled tomorrow."

    C. "No, I don't have constipation and don't need those stool softeners."

    D. "My granddaughter is such a big help to me. She makes sure my pills are right there in my pill container ready for me to take at the prescribed time."

60. Respiratory congestion during the dying phase is also known as

    A. Noisy breathing.

    B. Cheyne-Stokes respirations.

    C. Apnea.

    D. Kussmaul's respirations.

61. Which of the following is an effect of corticosteroids?

    A. Decreased anxiety

    B. Increased appetite

    C. Increased inflammation

    D. Increased somnolence

62. When a patient is comatose, the nurse should

    A. Speak to the patient as if he were not there.

    B. Speak to the patient as if he can hear.

    C. Do not speak in the room at all.

    D. Speak only to family members.

63. Nonpharmacological treatments for agitation

    A. Are rarely effective.

    B. Are only effective when used with psychotropic medications.

    C. Should not be directed by the family.

    D. Should always be used.

64. A patient has been receiving hydromorphone 15 mg by mouth every 4 hours. Because of his difficulty swallowing, he is being switched to IV morphine. What will his new per hour rate of morphine be?

    A. 0.83 mg/hour

    B. 3 mg/hour

    C. 5 mg/hour

    D. 46.9 mg/hour

65. When the patient dies in the home, the Schedule II drugs are

    A. Property of the hospice.

    B. Disposed of by the nurse with a witness present.

    C. Returned to the hospice or pharmacy for credit.

    D. Disposed of by the death vigil volunteer present at the time of the death.

66. A 4-year-old girl whose mother recently died is able to play with her friends, laugh, and enjoy her toys. She is

    A. Obviously depressed.

    B. Showing disrespect for her mother's memory.

    C. Grieving normally for a child her age.

    D. In need of intensive grief counseling.

67. A purpose for the hospice nurse to attend the death of a home hospice patient includes which of the following?

    A. Notification of family and friends.

    B. Completing the death certificate.

    C. Provision of comfort and support to the family.

    D. Prompt removal of medical equipment and supplies.

68. When communicating with a physician, the nurse's primary role is to

    A. Make her see the situation correctly.

    B. Carry out her orders.

    C. Advocate for the patient's wishes.

    D. Suggest an appropriate course of action.

69. Interdisciplinary collaborative practice in the hospice setting includes

    A. The coordination of patient care for other health providers.

    B. Interaction with interdisciplinary team members at time of admission.

    C. The understanding that the nurse case manager makes all of the decisions regarding the patient's care.

    D. The development of the plan of care in collaboration with the patient, family, other health and human service providers, and the interdisciplinary team.

70. The obligation to "do good" is

    A. Beneficence.

    B. Veracity.

    C. Nonmaleficence.

    D. Justice.

71. According to Medicare Hospice Benefit regulations, the 4 members of the core hospice services include

    A. Nurse, physician, medical social worker, and counseling.

    B. Nursing, hospice aide, chaplain, and volunteer.

    C. Whatever is needed to meet the care needs of the patient.

    D. Physician, patient, family, nurse.

72. The social worker and the palliative care nurse on the team do not agree on an approach to a family. The palliative care nurse's best response to this conflict would be to

    A. Contact the physician for orders.

    B. Become angry and walk away.

    C. Go to his supervisor to have her resolve the conflict.

    D. Work with the social worker directly to resolve the issue.

73. The importance of nursing research to palliative care and hospice is to

    A. Meet The Joint Commission requirements.

    B. Find a cure for cancer.

    C. Improve the care of persons with serious and life-threatening illness.

    D. Assure physicians will go along with the plan of care.

74. Hospice eligibility criteria for patients with late-stage human immunodeficiency virus (HIV) includes which of the following?

    A. CD4 count more than 25 cells/mm^3

    B. Advanced AIDS dementia complex

    C. Loss of at least 15% of lean body mass

    D. Central nervous system lymphoma

75. Treatment of seizures related to hypercalcemia includes which of the following?

    A. Glucagon

    B. Antibiotics

    C. Supplemental oxygen

    D. Oral and/or intravenous fluids

76. Which statement made by a patient indicates somatic pain?

    A. "I have a deep, dull ache on the side of my right thigh."

    B. "I have cramping all throughout my abdomen."

    C. "I have pain in my right shoulder though I don't remember injuring it."

    D. "It feels like a shock is going down my leg."

77. A benefit of nonsteroidal anti-inflammatory drugs includes all of the following **EXCEPT**

    A. Inhibit platelet aggregation.

    B. Antispasmodic.

    C. Analgesic.

    D. Antipyretic.

78. Type A chronic obstructive pulmonary disease (COPD) is emphysema. Which one of the following clinical features is the major symptom of emphysema?

    A. Dyspnea

    B. Productive cough

    C. Central cyanosis

    D. Weight gain

79. Calculate the lowest breakthrough dose of morphine for a patient who is on oral morphine 120 mg every 12 hours.

    A. 4 mg

    B. 8 mg

    C. 12 mg

    D. 24 mg

80. Dehydration is very common in the final phases of illness. Which of these statements is true about dehydration in the hospice patient? Dehydration is

    A. Often treated because the patient will be more comfortable.

    B. Never treated because it has advantages in the dying patient.

    C. Considered a medical emergency and is always treated.

    D. Most often not necessary to treat.

81. Advanced symptoms of end stage liver disease include all of the following **EXCEPT**

    A. Elevated albumin levels.

    B. Encephalopathy.

    C. Coagulopathy.

    D. Malnutrition.

82. "The state of adaptation in which exposure to a drug induces changes that result in a diminution of one or more of the drug's effects over time" is the definition of

    A. Addiction.

    B. Tolerance.

    C. Physical dependence.

    D. Pseudoaddiction.

83. When should a bowel regimen be initiated for patients taking opioids?

    A. After the patient has not experienced a bowel movement for 5 days

    B. When an enema is ineffective

    C. Upon initiation of the opioid

    D. When high fiber, fruits, and bulk foods have failed

84. Which statement most accurately describes dying patients and their families?

    A. A search for meaning and purpose in life is a common experience for dying patients and their families.

    B. Dying patients and their families are too consumed with financial problems ever to think about spiritual concerns.

    C. Dying patients and their families have little to fear because hospice takes care of everything.

    D. The same care plan can be used for all families because their needs are the same.

85. Hospice is

    A. Utilized when nothing more can be done.

    B. A philosophy of care to improve quality of life for the terminally ill persons and their families.

    C. A place where people go to be cared for as they die.

    D. Available to patients and families only on weekdays.

86. In 2014, palliative care was primarily delivered in the
    A. Home.
    B. Acute care setting.
    C. Nursing home.
    D. Rehabilitation setting.

87. How does hospice care differ when it is being paid for by a private insurance plan?
    A. The private insurance plans use a home health benefit for hospice.
    B. There are limits on the number of visits team members can make.
    C. The private insurance plan puts a dollar cap on services.
    D. The services must be the same if the hospice is Medicare certified.

88. Which side effects of chemotherapy can be asymptomatic but have serious life-threatening potential?
    A. Bone marrow suppression.
    B. Epithelial denudement of the gastrointestinal tract
    C. Bone marrow suppression—especially the red cells—making the patient susceptible to anemia
    D. Anorexia and weight loss

89. The prognostic eligibility requirements for palliative and hospice care are
    A. A 6-month prognosis for both.
    B. A 6-month prognosis for hospice and prognostic estimate for palliative care.
    C. Not applicable to hospice or palliative care.
    D. Directly related to functional status for both hospice and palliative care.

90. The focus of palliative care is
    A. The patient and family as the unit of care.
    B. The patient as the unit of care.
    C. On symptoms as the unit of care.
    D. On reimbursement.

91. It is inappropriate to suggest aggressive curative treatment when
    A. Cure is possible.
    B. There is a realistic chance of worthwhile prolongation of life.
    C. The side effects of the treatment are more distressing than the potential benefits.
    D. A patient chooses a clinical trial with informed consent.

92. Abstinence syndrome
    A. Happens mainly with opioids with a short half-life.
    B. Is another term for myoclonus.
    C. Occurs when an opioid is abruptly stopped.
    D. Symptoms include sedation.

93. A benefit of using lorazepam over zolpidem to treat insomnia is that lorazepam
    A. Produces less rebound insomnia.
    B. Has a decreased risk of dependency.
    C. Is also effective at reducing anxiety.
    D. Produces less drowsiness upon awakening.

94. A patient is taking his breakthrough pain medication 6 times per day. Which of the following is the appropriate action for the nurse to take? Suggest an increase in the
    A. Amount of the breakthrough dose.
    B. Amount of the scheduled dose.
    C. Frequency of the breakthrough dose.
    D. Frequency of the scheduled dose.

95. Lymphedema
    A. Can be an effect of chemotherapy.
    B. Can be treated with lymphatic massage.
    C. Is a common symptom of cirrhosis.
    D. Responds well to diuretics.

96. Of the following cancers, which has the best 5-year survival rate in the United States?
    A. Colorectal
    B. Esophageal
    C. Hepatocellular
    D. Pancreatic

97. Which of the following is a true statement regarding barriers to pain management?
    A. Fears about addiction persist.
    B. Instruction on pain during basic nursing education is adequate.
    C. Regulations do not impede pain management.
    D. Use of 0–10 scale is adequate to assess pain.

98. Patients with the following diagnoses are most at risk for hemorrhage **EXCEPT**

    A. Advanced laryngeal cancer.

    B. Hepatic failure.

    C. Multiple myeloma.

    D. Pancytopenia.

99. A 70-year-old woman has been cared for by her son and daughter-in-law in their home for the 2 years since her debilitating stroke. She is now receiving home hospice care for an aggressive cancer. In talking with the son, the nurse discovers that he thinks they are doing a "horrible job" caring for his mother. No signs of abuse or neglect have been noted. Which of the following is the best initial response the nurse could make?

    A. "Has your wife not been helping care for your mother?"

    B. "I'll arrange for the hospice aide to come more often."

    C. "You have been doing a great job caring for your mother for over 2 years, but I do think that it's time to transfer your mother to a nursing home."

    D. "I bet this has been hard for you and your wife—you've cared for your mother a long time and feeling overwhelmed is common. Can you tell me more about what you're feeling?"

100. Allodynia is

    A. Increasing pain despite treatment.

    B. Pain from a stimulus that does not usually cause pain.

    C. Painful muscle twitching.

    D. Pain from nerve involvement.

101. Which of the following is a reversible cause of anorexia/cachexia syndrome (ACS) in end stage illness?

    A. Xerostomia

    B. Peritoneal carcinomatosis

    C. Increasing catabolism

    D. Chemotherapy

102. The only child of a stable patient with end stage cancer needs to have a surgical procedure that will not allow her to care for her mother on hospice care for 4 days. What level of hospice care is appropriate for the patient while the caregiver has the surgery and recuperates from it?

    A. Continuous care

    B. General inpatient care

    C. Respite care

    D. Routine home care

103. Which patient is the most appropriate for administration of rectal analgesics? A patient with

   A. Anorectal pain.

   B. Chronic leukemia.

   C. Disseminated intravascular coagulation (DIC).

   D. Nausea and vomiting.

104. The following are underlying causes of fatigue **EXCEPT**

   A. Extreme heat or cold.

   B. Hyperglycemia.

   C. Hypocalcemia.

   D. Hypoxia.

105. Gabapentin

   A. Is an antidepressant.

   B. Is effective for neuropathic pain.

   C. Requires lower doses than pregabalin.

   D. Should not be used in patients with renal failure.

106. A physical modality for pain relief that involves "life force energy" is

   A. Reiki.

   B. Acupressure.

   C. Transcutaneous nerve stimulation.

   D. Massage.

107. The staff of an assisted living facility calls the hospice nurse to report a new onset of confusion resulting in a fall in an active, independent, and afebrile 90-year-old hospice patient with chronic leukemia. What is the likely underlying cause of the confusion and fall?

   A. Dementia

   B. Nearing death awareness

   C. Progression of her leukemia

   D. Urinary tract infection

108. All of the following are challenges to providing palliative care to homeless patients **EXCEPT**
    A. Homeless patients have a shorter life expectance than those who are not homeless.
    B. Most homeless persons report having multiple chronic conditions.
    C. Receiving healthcare at emergency departments does not improve the overall health of homeless persons.
    D. Social service income support is usually only available to those with dependent children living in low-income households.

109. A patient with a rapidly progressing disease refuses pain medication because "my culture does not permit anything to lessen suffering." Which of the following would be the best response?
    A. "At this time in your life you would be permitted pain medication."
    B. "I cannot let you be in pain."
    C. "I would like to learn more about your culture."
    D. "No culture wants people to be in pain."

110. What is the first step in the assessment of new onset diarrhea in a patient who uses dietary fiber?
    A. Collect a stool sample to rule out *Clostridium difficile*.
    B. Assess for a recent initiation of opioids for pain.
    C. Perform a digital rectal exam to rule out impaction.
    D. Order an abdominal x-ray to rule out a complete bowel obstruction.

111. In all of the following situations abuse should be suspected and immediate action taken **EXCEPT**
    A. A wife does not allow her husband, the patient, to speak to the hospice nurse without her being present.
    B. Bruises on the patient are explained by falls when the nurse has not witnessed an unsteady gate.
    C. During a morning home visit, a patient with progressive Alzheimer's disease is found to be incontinent. She tells the nurse her son refuses to help her to the bathroom at night.
    D. Reports by the nursing assistant as he was leaving a home that he overheard the caregiver angrily tell the patient to stop reporting her pain to everyone.

112. Hypnosis
    A. Cannot be done by the patient.
    B. Has not been proven to be of benefit in the management of pain.
    C. Is a technique to enhance the mind's ability to affect the physical body.
    D. Uses energy fields to promote comfort and/or symptom relief.

113. Which of the following is true about typical angina? Typical angina

    A. Decreases as people age.

    B. Is not always a symptom of inadequate blood flow to the heart muscle.

    C. Is rarely life-threatening.

    D. Is usually relieved by rest in 5 minutes.

114. Medicare Hospice Benefit recertifications

    A. Are available for an unlimited number of 60-day periods.

    B. Are only available to patients living in their own home.

    C. Require a physician or nurse practitioner to have a face-to-face encounter with the patient starting with the third rectification period.

    D. Use stricter criteria than initial certification.

115. Which of the following is true about pain management for patients with serious and persistent mental illness?

    A. Analgesics are not needed if the patient is taking an antidepressant.

    B. Opioid analgesics cannot be used due to interactions with antipsychotics.

    C. Pain does not increase the risk of suicide.

    D. Studies have indicated that pain is undertreated in people with a history of psychiatric disorders.

116. Extrapyramidal symptoms (EPS) are a common symptom of which disease?

    A. Amyotropic lateral sclerosis (ALS)

    B. Chronic obstructive pulmonary disease (COPD)

    C. Multiple myeloma

    D. Parkinson's disease

117. Syndrome of inappropriate secretion of antidiuretic hormone (SIADH) is

    A. Diagnosed in part by urine osmolality higher than plasma osmolality.

    B. Primarily associated with renal cancer.

    C. The inappropriate production and secretion of the antidiuretic hormone causing hypernatremia.

    D. Treated by encouraging fluid intake.

118. For a minimally conscious patient in the final days of life in which pain is suspected, which is the best method of determining if the patient does have pain?

    A. A furrowed brow.

    B. A trail of an analgesic.

    C. Vocalization during turning.

    D. Unconscious patients do not feel pain.

119. Which of the following medications does not lower the seizure threshold?

    A. Chlorpromazine

    B. Haloperidol

    C. Nortriptyline

    D. Tramadol

120. A 92-year-old cognitively intact patient is being admitted to hospice with advanced metastatic breast cancer. She admits to the hospice nurse that neither she nor her husband are able to read and she does not know what medications she should be taking. What would be the best way for the nurse to help the patient understand her medication regimen?

    A. Ask her what would be the best way for her to remember her medications.

    B. Have a member of the team come every day to fill her pillbox.

    C. Make her repeat it back to the nurse until she has it correct.

    D. Use pictures of medications taped to a list.

121. Which of the following is an indication of an aggressively progressing lymphoma?

    A. Bony lytic lesions

    B. Lynch syndrome

    C. Presence of *BRCA2* gene

    D. T-cell origin

122. What is the most common symptom at end of life regardless of underlying disease?

    A. Dyspnea

    B. Fatigue

    C. Noisy breathing

    D. Pain

123. A patient with a large laceration on her arm from a fall is being seen in a palliative care clinic. The laceration will require her caregiver to change the dressing at home. Even though he has been taught the dressing change and was able to demonstrate it for the nurse, the caregiver is worried that he will not remember the steps and wants to be able to watch an online video on dressing changes. What recommendation regarding caregiving online videos should the nurse give the caregiver?

    A. Look on the dressing manufacturer's website for a video.

    B. Make sure that he has the correct name of the dressing change to search.

    C. Tell him that large university hospital websites have many online teaching materials.

    D. The nurse should watch any video before recommending them to a caregiver.

124. Volunteer service hours must account for what percent of all direct patient care hours if the hospice is Medicare certified?

    A. 1%

    B. 5%

    C. 8%

    D. 10%

125. During an initial assessment, the patient reports dyspnea and on physical exam, the nurse notes stony dullness with percussion on the entire lower left side. This is likely due to

    A. Aspiration pneumonia.

    B. Chronic bronchitis.

    C. Metastatic lesion in the lung.

    D. Pleural effusion.

126. A patient with American College of Cardiology/American Heart Association (ACC/AHA) stage D heart failure tells the nurse he is planning a trip to Alaska with his family a year from now. What is the nurse's best response?

    A. "You won't be living next year; you must accept that."

    B. "Your disease is at a stage you can expect to be able to travel."

    C. "We can arrange to have a hospice program take care of you in Alaska."

    D. "What do you understand about your illness?"

Practice Exam Answers

1. Answer is B (2B6)

    A. Incorrect: This symptom is suggestive of the acute dying phase.

    B. **Correct:** Myoclonus is a symptom of the toxic effects of morphine metabolites.

    C. Incorrect: Respiratory depression causing *hypo*ventilation may be a significant acute symptom of opioid excess.

    D. Incorrect: Periodic apnea reflects neurologic changes with active dying; diaphoresis may occur with temperature change or increased pain, infection, or anxiety.

2. Answer is B (1B1)

    A. Incorrect: Lung commonly metastasizes to bone.

    B. **Correct:** Colorectal mainly metastasizes to the liver, lung, and peritoneum.

    C. Incorrect: Prostate commonly metastasizes to bone.

    D. Incorrect: Breast commonly metastasizes to bone.

3. Answer is D (3C3)

    A. Incorrect: Meperidine should not be used in end stage diseases. In addition, normeperidine is a neurologic toxic metabolite of meperidine and accumulates even with small doses.

    B. Incorrect: Lorazepam is indicated for anxiety, which is not the etiology of air hunger in this case.

    C. Incorrect: While it may help to open the airways, it has no direct effect on the sensation of air hunger.

    D. **Correct:** Opioids provide palliative support for symptoms of breathlessness or suffocation.

4. Answer is C (1B3)

    A. Incorrect: This would be unnecessary if it was determined that the patient's dyspnea has a reversible cause.

    B. Incorrect: Holding all medications would not be the first step and may make the dyspnea worse.

    C. **Correct:** First, conduct a complete assessment that includes the patient's reports of adherence with her medication schedule.

    D. Incorrect: As there may be other etiologic reasons, this would not be an appropriate action.

5. Answer is B (3D7)

    A. Incorrect: Although some medications can cause these symptoms (e.g., opioids, vincristine), this is most likely not the cause.

    B. **Correct:** The classic symptoms of bowel obstruction are constipation, distension, abdominal discomfort, and vomiting.

    C. Incorrect: Classic symptoms of spinal cord compression are back pain, urinary incontinence, and changes in reflexes.

    D. Incorrect: This patient had no respiratory symptoms such as dyspnea, chest pain, fever, or cough.

6. Answer is C (3D7)

    A. Incorrect: A nasogastric (NG) tube would prevent vomiting and therefore provide comfort.

    B. Incorrect: Corticosteroids can relieve obstruction especially if caused by metastatic disease progression.

    C. **Correct:** Metoclopramide would have no value for a patient with an obstruction.

    D. Incorrect: Octreotide can reverse symptoms of small bowel obstruction.

7. Answer is A (3K3)

    A. **Correct:** This would be an important option. A quiet atmosphere with limited stimulation would be preferred in this situation.

    B. Incorrect: Passive range of motion would most likely be very painful for him.

    C. Incorrect: While music therapy can sometimes be soothing, in this case, frequent stimulation would not be advisable.

    D. Incorrect: Involve and support the family whenever possible.

8. Answer is D (1A)

    A. Incorrect: There would be no reason to sedate him. His family needs reassurance and support as well as education to help them understand what is happening.

    B. Incorrect: Restraints would be very inappropriate and may cause agitation.

    C. Incorrect: While there is a spiritual aspect to this situation, the action of choice is to recognize the normalcy of what is happening.

    D. **Correct:** "Seeing" people who have died is common and should not be considered confusion. Near-death awareness manifests itself in many ways. Near-death awareness is associated with dreams or visions of deceased people, God, or heaven/afterlife; acceptance of mortality may be revealed through talks of a trip or a journey or fear of being alone.

9. Answer is B (1B1)

    A. Incorrect: While facial edema and dyspnea can be a sign of an allergy, bluish edematous arms are not likely to be related to an allergic reaction to morphine. Allergic responses usually include pruritus and skin flushing.

    B. **Correct:** These are classic signs of superior vena cava syndrome (SVCS), an oncologic emergency requiring immediate attention.

    C. Incorrect: Signs of heart failure include edema but normally of the lower extremities.

    D. Incorrect: Pneumonia does not cause edematous arms and face.

10. Answer is D (4D3)

    A. Incorrect: Mourning is the cultural response to having suffered a loss.

    B. Incorrect: Grief is the process of psychological, social, and somatic reactions to a perceived loss.

    C. Incorrect: Bereavement is the state of having suffered a loss.

    D. **Correct:** This is the definition of anticipatory grief.

11. Answer is A (1B8)

    A. **Correct:** A change in the patient's behavior (in this case, the resident's usual behavior of wandering in the hallway) is considered the gold standard for determining the presence of pain in someone with dementia who cannot self-report.

    B. Incorrect: While nursing assistants know the resident well and can provide valuable information, it is the resident's change in behavior that is the best indicator.

    C. Incorrect: While the blood pressure can increase with acute pain, frequent monitoring of the blood pressure of a patient with dementia is not ideal.

    D. Incorrect: Though the person's self-report of pain is preferable, people with dementia may not be able to reliably use a pain scale.

12. Answer is D (1A)

    A. Incorrect: Inability to sleep is not seen in the imminently dying. Quite the opposite is true. The dying person may sleep most of the time due to decreasing cerebral perfusion and metabolic changes.

    B. Incorrect: Senses, specifically sight, hearing, touch, smell, and taste decline significantly in the imminently dying.

    C. Incorrect: Low blood pressure with a weak and irregular pulse is seen frequently in the imminently dying due to failing cardiac contractions.

    D. **Correct:** Dysphagia appears to be a common symptom in the end stages of many diseases probably due to muscle weakness and loss of gag and swallowing reflexes.

13. Answer is C (2A1)

    A. Incorrect: Liquid morphine is immediate release and can be used for relief of pain but a thorough assessment must be performed first.

    B. Incorrect: Sustained release morphine is a long acting medication and is usually dosed once the amount of medication required to relieve the pain is determined. Severe pain should be initially dosed with a short-acting opioid formulation.

    C. **Correct:** The patient needs to be quickly assessed with a review of her history prior to calling the physician for the appropriate medication order.

    D. Incorrect: The assessment must be completed first before calling the physician for appropriate orders.

14. Answer is B (2C2)
    A. Incorrect: The pharmacological interventions are not replaced by nonpharmacological interventions.
    B. **Correct:** The nonpharmacological interventions often can augment pharmacological management.
    C. Incorrect: Pain relief requires pharmacological interventions; family needs to be educated to understand pain management.
    D. Incorrect: Optimal pain management should never be a matter of provider convenience.

15. Answer is B (3G4)
    A. Incorrect: Stage I is when the skin is deep pink, red, or mottled.
    B. **Correct:** Stage II is when the skin is blistered, cracked, or abraded.
    C. Incorrect: Stage III is when there is a craterlike wound with involvement of the underlying tissues.
    D. Incorrect: Stage IV is when deep ulceration, necrosis, or wet/dry black exudate is present.

16. Answer is C (4D2)
    A. Incorrect: Mourning is the cultural response to having suffered a loss.
    B. Incorrect: Grief is the process of psychological, social, and somatic reactions to a perceived loss.
    C. **Correct:** This is the definition of bereavement.
    D. Incorrect: Anticipatory grief is the process of psychological, social, and somatic reactions to a perceived future loss.

17. Answer is B (1B1)
    A. Incorrect: This describes tumor lysis syndrome. Disseminated intravascular coagulation (DIC) is inappropriate and exaggerated overstimulation of normal coagulation when thrombosis then bleeding occurs.
    B. **Correct:** These are signs and symptoms of DIC. Other symptoms include acrocyanosis, frank gangrene, altered sensation, ulceration of gastrointestinal system, decreased urinary output, and dyspnea.
    C. Incorrect: This is the treatment for superior vena cava syndrome. Treatment for DIC includes management of underlying cause, oxygen, fluid replacement; consider blood products if appropriate, and anticoagulant.
    D. Incorrect: While DIC can occur in patients with acute leukemia, it does not occur in the other conditions. This is describing cardiac tamponade. DIC most commonly occurs in patients with sepsis, acute leukemia, tumor lysis, massive tissue injury, obstetric complications, and transfusion reactions.

18. Answer is B (3A2)

    A. Incorrect: An assessment should be done to determine the best food consistency for this patient.

    B. **Correct:** As he is having difficulty swallowing, oral hygiene is very important to prevent complications such as mouth soreness and infections.

    C. Incorrect: With his short prognosis, a swallowing study would not be indicated.

    D. Incorrect: Lemon adds to the mouth dryness and can be painful if there are inflamed areas secondary to radiation. Glycerin has an alcohol base and ultimately worsens dryness.

19. Answer is A (6A1)

    A. **Correct:** The interdisciplinary team must focus on symptom management as a top priority. All other domains respond positively when physical symptoms are alleviated.

    B. Incorrect: Problems must be prioritized and coordinated among the team.

    C. Incorrect: Spiritual pain may present in any of the domains.

    D. Incorrect: All members of the interdisciplinary team are vital. None are more important than others.

20. Answer is C (1B8)

    A. Incorrect: Individuals with advanced dementia should have minimal stimulation.

    B. Incorrect: Healthcare providers should use simple words and explanations for the person with dementia.

    C. **Correct:** Safety is a priority with persons with dementia. Supervision, minimal stimulation, and discouraging sleep during daytime hours maximize night safety.

    D. Incorrect: Naps should be discouraged at any time during daytime hours.

21. Answer is A (3G1)

    A. **Correct:** Xerostomia is dry mouth and can be a side effect of medications and a long-term effect of radiation therapy.

    B. Incorrect: Stomatitis is inflammation of the oral cavity and is not usually caused by these medications.

    C. Incorrect: Dysphagia is difficulty swallowing and is not usually associated as a side effect of these medications; it is common during and directly after radiation.

    D. Incorrect: Esophagitis is inflammation of the esophageal lining and is not usually associated with these medications; it is common during and directly after radiation therapy.

22. Answer is C (5C5)

   A. Incorrect: Healthcare providers have an obligation to honor the patient's wishes as written in the advance directive.

   B. Incorrect: The advance directive must be respected but a discussion needs to also occur with his sister to assist and support her concerns while educating about the patient's wishes.

   C. **Correct:** Since the advance directive was completed when the patient was decisional, it must be respected. Discussing these issues with his sister may help her to recognize these are the wishes of her brother.

   D. Incorrect: Aggressive care is inappropriate in this situation and is against the stated wishes of the patient.

23. Answer is D (4C1)

   A. Incorrect: Spiritual care must be provided according to the patient's religious preferences, if he/she has a religious preference.

   B. Incorrect: Spiritual care can be provided by anyone.

   C. Incorrect: Spiritual care is provided according to the wishes of the patient. While spiritual care is offered to all hospice patients, if they do not wish to have spiritual counseling, it is not required.

   D. **Correct:** Spiritual care is intended to relieve the spiritual suffering of the patient and family.

24. Answer is A (4D2)

   A. **Correct:** Grief is the feelings related to the perception of the loss.

   B. Incorrect: Grief is feelings, not an overt expression.

   C. Incorrect: Although the expression of grief differs among ethnic groups, the definition does not reflect ethnic expressions.

   D. Incorrect: This definition refers to the mood state of grief, which consists of variable levels of sadness.

25. Answer is D (5C)

   A. Incorrect: This is 1 method of working toward improved access to care and community resources by influencing or formulating health and social policy.

   B. Incorrect: Working for better insurance coverage is an example of advocating for the patient.

   C. Incorrect: The nurse should speak up when the team's recommendations are not within the patient's best interest.

   D. **Correct:** This is not advocating for the patient's wishes and preferences.

26. Answer is A (7B1)

   A. **Correct:** A usually long-term relationship between an experienced person (mentor) and a less experienced person (mentee), in the example of a hospice and/or palliative care nurse, in which clinical and professional issues are discussed and dealt with.

   B. Incorrect: This describes role modeling.

   C. Incorrect: This describes precepting.

   D. Incorrect: This is part of the definition of peer review.

27. Answer is D (6A2)

   A. Incorrect: Review of the care plan is an aspect of supervision.

   B. Incorrect: Observation of care being given is an aspect of supervision.

   C. Incorrect: Documentation of the supervisory visit is part of the supervision.

   D. **Correct:** As the feeling of a high work burden is connected to job dissatisfaction, decreased job commitment, and turnover, the supervisor should listen to the nursing assistant's concerns. It needs to be noted that a supervisor should not tell anyone what to "feel."

28. Answer is A (5A3)

   A. **Correct:** This change would be most beneficial for patient and family.

   B. Incorrect: Providing assistance will allow the wife to get needed rest.

   C. Incorrect: Teaching his wife how to make an occupied bed and how to give a bed bath would not be necessary in this situation.

   D. Incorrect: There is no evidence that his fatigue and spending more time in bed are related to his pain medication.

29. Answer is B (5C4)

   A. Incorrect: The patient would not benefit from strengthening exercises at this stage nor would he most likely be able to tolerate them.

   B. **Correct:** It is appropriate to ask if a visit is needed from a team member before initiating the request. Asking them separately acknowledges that they may have different needs.

   C. Incorrect: While the deterioration of his status could bring up many spiritual issues, it is appropriate to ask if either would like to talk to the hospice chaplain.

   D. Incorrect: There is no need for a hospice patient to go to his attending physician's office. If he needs to be seen by a physician, a provider can go to the home.

30. Answer is D (7B2)

    A. **Incorrect:** Confidentiality is the patient's right to maintain privacy regarding personal and medical matters.

    B. **Incorrect:** Autonomy is an individual's personal liberty.

    C. **Incorrect:** Beneficence is the duty to help others.

    D. **Correct:** Justice is to consider rules and actions that result in fair and equitable use of available resources.

31. Answer is C (7A8)

    A. Incorrect: See C.

    B. Incorrect: See C.

    C. **Correct:** The correct benefit periods are 90-, 90-, and unlimited 60-day periods.

    D. Incorrect: See C.

32. Answer is B (7B4)

    A. **Incorrect:** In many situations, this activity would be within professional boundaries.

    B. **Correct:** This example would definitely overstep the professional boundaries between the nurse and patient/family.

    C. **Incorrect:** This activity would be well within one's professional boundaries.

    D. **Incorrect:** This activity would be within professional boundaries as long as the patient requested it as indicated and the team member feels comfortable praying.

33. Answer is B (5C3)

    A. **Incorrect:** This response would be unprofessional and unacceptable.

    B. **Correct:** Professionalism requires open communication with the nurse's assigned supervisor. Expressing concerns is important to maintaining open communication and trust.

    C. **Incorrect:** Effective, open communication is necessary to maintain trust and effective management. The direct supervisor should appreciate open communication and honesty with the staff.

    D. **Incorrect:** This behavior is unprofessional and unacceptable.

34. Answer is A (3B3)

    A. **Correct:** Repeated blood pressure readings taken in the lying, sitting, and standing positions would provide sufficient information to make a determination whether the antihypertensive medications could be decreased or discontinued. With end stage disease, blood pressure naturally decreases eliminating the need for continuing antihypertensive medications. The syncopal responses are often related to orthostatic hypotension.

    B. Incorrect: Although safety is a concern with this patient, she should not be encouraged to remain in bed. Education of patient and family should include the importance of having help when getting up.

    C. Incorrect: Fluids are very important to prevent syncopal reactions. Dehydration is also a common cause of orthostatic hypotension.

    D. Incorrect: Restraining any patient for any reason is inappropriate. Restraints cause a higher percentage of deaths and injury.

35. Answer is A (4A2)

    A. **Correct:** The patient's goals determine the plan of care.

    B. Incorrect: It is inappropriate for the physician to try once more for a cure if the patient does not want it.

    C. Incorrect: The patient is the center of decision-making. Decisions to initiate therapies should not be done in response to the demands of the family.

    D. Incorrect: The decision to institute therapy should be in accordance to the patient's wishes and according to the plan of care.

36. Answer is B (6B3)

    A. Incorrect: The current Medicare Hospice election does not remain valid if the patient revokes the Medicare Hospice Benefit.

    B. **Correct:** The patient will lose the remaining days of the current period if they revoke the Medicare Hospice Benefit.

    C. Incorrect: Only the patient (or patient's representative) may revoke the Medicare Hospice Benefit.

    D. Incorrect: The patient can always come back to the Medicare Hospice Benefit as long as they meet the criteria.

37. Answer is B (2D1)

    A. Incorrect: Respiratory depression is a side effect, but tolerance develops rapidly to respiratory depression, however, it is not dose limiting.

    B. **Correct:** Myoclonus is the chronic spasm of a muscle; if myoclonus is present, accepted practice is to rotate to another opioid.

    C. Incorrect: Constipation is experienced in all patients receiving opioids and should be anticipated.

    D. Incorrect: Dehydration is not a side effect of opioids.

38. Answer is B (3B2)

    A. Incorrect: His decision-making capacity now is the main concern to move forward with his plan of care.

    B. **Correct:** His decision-making capacity needs to be determined. If he were deemed to be able to make decisions, he would speak for himself. If not, his healthcare proxy and/or advanced directive would be used to direct care according to his wishes.

    C. Incorrect: Decision-making capacity must be determined first.

    D. Incorrect: Although the daughter is the next of kin, the patient's wishes, if known, must be honored.

39. Answer is B (4C1)

    A. Incorrect: This is important, but not the first priority.

    B. **Correct:** Knowing how the family makes decisions and who the decision makers are is priority.

    C. Incorrect: This is important, but not the first priority.

    D. Incorrect: This is important, but not the first priority.

40. Answer is C (3G4)

    A. Incorrect: Surgical repair would be used on stage IV wounds only.

    B. Incorrect: Irrigation and debridement is the therapy for stage III wounds.

    C. **Correct:** The therapy for stage II wounds is to relieve pressure and apply protective/occlusive dressings.

    D. Incorrect: Applying protective dressings is the correct choice. A & D ointment would not be considered appropriate in this case.

41. Answer is A (2B4)

    $100 \times 3 = 300$

    $10 \times 6 = 60$

    $300 + 60 = 360$

    $360 \div 30 = 12$

    $12 \times 20 = 240$

    $240 \div 6 = 40$ mg every 4 hours

42. Answer is C (1B2)

   A. Incorrect: Artificial nutrition may be needed as the disease progresses, but respiratory failure is the usual cause of death.

   B. Incorrect: While aspiration leading to pneumonia is a possibility, respiratory failure is the usual cause of death.

   C. **Correct:** Respiratory failure from progressive muscle weakness is the usual cause of death.

   D. Incorrect: Cholinergic crisis occurs in patients with myasthenia gravis after taking too much anticholinergic medication.

43. Answer is B (1B5)

   A. Incorrect: Less than one-third of patients with end stage renal disease have completed an advance directive.

   B. **Correct:** Patients with chronic renal failure cannot be seeking dialysis or renal transplant, or are discontinuing dialysis.

   C. Incorrect: Morphine should be avoided in patients with chronic renal failure. Fentanyl and methadone are better choices.

   D. Incorrect: Cognitive impairment results from uremia.

44. Answer is A (2B5)

   A. **Correct:** The anticholinergic side effects of tricyclic antidepressants can cause constipation. Diarrhea is not a major side effect of tricyclic antidepressants.

   B. Incorrect: Tricyclic antidepressants can cause urinary retention.

   C. Incorrect: Tricyclic antidepressants can cause myoclonus.

   D. Incorrect: Tricyclic antidepressants can lower seizure threshold.

45. Answer is A (5C2)

   A. **Correct:** Trying to determine what the patient will say limits the ability to listen to what they are saying.

   B. Incorrect: Even though some topics can be very upsetting to talk about, the patient would not be talking about it if he/she did not want to.

   C. Incorrect: While there are points that need communicated to patients (e.g., education, changes to the plan), patients should be able to direct the conversation.

   D. Incorrect: Silence can give patients time to think about what they said and if they want to talk anymore at this time.

46. Answer is B (3H11)
    A. Incorrect: There is no indication that there is a change in his mood or how he is coping.
    B. **Correct:** Any thoughts of suicide or a desire to hasten death need to be assessed immediately.
    C. Incorrect: There is no indication that there is a change in his mood or how he is coping.
    D. Incorrect: While expressions of anger can mean many things and needs to be investigated further, his wish to hasten death should be explored immediately.

47. Answer is D (4C1)
    A. Incorrect: It cannot be assumed that she follows this custom of her culture. The patient should decide who attends the meetings.
    B. Incorrect: Inviting only the patient does not allow other alternatives of who could attend.
    C. Incorrect: It would be unethical to not tell her about the meeting.
    D. **Correct:** Asking who she wants to attend gives her control. It cannot be assumed that she follows this custom of her culture.

48. Answer is B (4D1)
    A. Incorrect: This question is leading the patient. See B.
    B. **Correct:** Life review is about finding meaning and reflecting on memories of life events.
    C. Incorrect: This question is leading the patient. See B.
    D. Incorrect: This question is leading the patient. See B.

49. Answer is A (7B7)
    A. **Correct:** While compassion fatigue can lead to burnout, it is not one of its components. Compassion fatigue is almost identical to posttraumatic stress disorder, except that it applies to those emotionally affected by the trauma of another (usually a client or family member).
    B. Incorrect: Cynicism and depersonalization, a component of burnout, is negative, callous, or an excessively detached response to various aspects of the job. It is closely related to exhaustion and both result in distancing oneself from work.
    C. Incorrect: Emotional exhaustion, a component of burnout, is feelings of being over-extended and depleted of one's emotional and physical resources.
    D. Incorrect: Ineffectiveness and lack of personal accomplishment, a component of burnout, are feelings of incompetence and a lack of achievement and productivity at work. Ineffectiveness and lack of personal accomplishment may be experienced along with emotional exhaustion and cynicism.

50. Answer is B (2B4)

    $2.5 \times 24 = 60$

    $60 \div 10 = 6$

    $6 \times 30 = 180$

    $180 \div 6 = 30$ mg every 4 hours

51. Answer is B (1B1)

    A. Incorrect: See B.

    B. **Correct:** Toxicity to the cardiac system induced by chemotherapy is similar in presentation to congestive heart failure with dyspnea, cough, pedal edema, and poor response to diuretics or digitalis (most common with anthracyclines).

    C. Incorrect: See B.

    D. Incorrect: See B.

52. Answer is D (2A1)

    A. Incorrect: Many people with chronic conditions learn the medical terms associated with their condition.

    B. Incorrect: People with chronic pain can enjoy activities even when they are in pain.

    C. Incorrect: While resting may help his back pain, he has chosen to continue to sit and play cards.

    D. **Correct:** Long periods of sitting are painful for those with chronic back pain. The pain medication will allow him to continue to enjoy the card game.

53. Answer is C (1B9)

    A. Incorrect: With relatively stable diabetes and organ failure, glucose monitoring will be needed when a decision about the management of her diabetes is needed.

    B. Incorrect: With relatively stable diabetes and organ failure, her insulin will most likely be decreased especially with renal failure.

    C. **Correct:** Glucose testing can determine if the often vague symptoms of hypoglycemia are hypoglycemia so it can be treated, and thus lead to enhanced quality of life.

    D. Incorrect: Hb A_1C levels are usually not needed once organ failure develops.

54. Answer is C (2A2)

    A. Incorrect: Hyperalgesia is common central pain or post stroke pain.

    B. Incorrect: Pain associated with deconditioning is common in patients with amyotrophic lateral sclerosis.

    C. **Correct:** Painful spasms are common in patients with multiple sclerosis as well as paroxysmal trigeminal neuralgia, optic neuritis, periorbital pain, extremity pain, including dysesthesia, allodynia, and painful electric shock sensations.

    D. Incorrect: Visceral pain is common in patients with sickle cell disease.

55. Answer is D (2A4)

　　A. Incorrect: Asking a Veteran about specific experiences from his time in the military is inappropriate. If he wants to talk, he will.

　　B. Incorrect: It is unethical to give any medication without the patient's knowledge.

　　C. Incorrect: While he may have spiritual issues and appreciate a visit from the chaplain, he should be asked first as he asked to be left alone.

　　D. **Correct:** Acknowledging that he has a painful condition and informing him about available analgesics is the best choice.

56. Answer is B (1B1)

　　A. Incorrect: See B.

　　B. **Correct:** Brachytherapy is a radioactive source that is placed inside of or directly on the body.

　　C. Incorrect: See B.

　　D. Incorrect: See B.

57. Answer is C (2B3)

　　A. Incorrect: 325 mg is half the adult single dose.

　　B. Incorrect: 1000 mg is 2 extra strength tablets.

　　C. **Correct:** This is the maximum daily recommended allowance of acetaminophen for an older individual.

　　D. Incorrect: 4000 mg per day is the previous recommended per day total.

58. Answer is C (2B1)

　　A. Incorrect: Visceral pain requires opioids. It is squeezing, cramping pain of internal organs, soft tissues, or bone.

　　B. Incorrect: Somatic pain is aching, throbbing pain experienced in organs, soft tissues, or bones and benefits from opioids.

　　C. **Correct:** Neuropathic pain is generally due to damage to the nervous system. Adjuvants are often used to enhance the analgesic efficacy of opioids especially in cases of neuropathic pain. Antidepressants, anticonvulsants, and corticosteroids are examples of adjuvants useful in treating neuropathic pain.

　　D. Incorrect: Referred pain is a type of visceral pain.

59. Answer is C (2D1)

　　A.　Incorrect: A pain rating of 2–3 indicates that the patient's pain is well controlled and she is taking her pain medication regularly.

　　B.　Incorrect: Taking 4 tablets per day would mean this person had 2 more days left in her supply. Filling the prescription should occur soon.

　　C.　**Correct:** Constipation is an expected side effect of opioids and having no signs of constipation could make one suspicious of opioid diversion.

　　D.　Incorrect: Family guiding medication administration is very helpful and indicates a concerned family member caregiver.

60. Answer is A (3C1)

　　A.　**Correct:** Terminal secretions are caused by respiratory congestion during the dying phase. The less preferred term for noisy breathing is death rattle.

　　B.　Incorrect: Cheyne-Stokes is an irregular pattern of breathing commonly associated with the dying process.

　　C.　Incorrect: Apnea is the absence of respirations.

　　D.　Incorrect: Kussmaul's respirations are deep, rapid respiratory patterns seen in coma or diabetic ketoacidosis.

61. Answer is B (2B5)

　　A.　Incorrect: Anxiety is an effect of corticosteroids.

　　B.　**Correct:** Corticosteroids can increase the patient's appetite.

　　C.　Incorrect: Decreased inflammation is an effect of corticosteroids.

　　D.　Incorrect: Insomnia is an effect of corticosteroids.

62. Answer is B (3A3)

　　A.　Incorrect: Comatose persons can hear—especially familiar sounds; therefore, family and healthcare providers should be encouraged to continue to speak to the patient in soft soothing tones.

　　B.　**Correct:** One should continue to speak as if the patient hears as it is believed the sense of hearing is the last sense to leave.

　　C.　Incorrect: Patients are comforted by familiar sounds—it is important to continue to speak softly.

　　D.　Incorrect: Patient can likely still hear.

63. Answer is D (3K1)

    A. Incorrect: Nonpharmacological treatments for agitation can be effective.

    B. Incorrect: Nonpharmacological treatments for agitation can be effective regardless of whether or not the patient is taking psychotropic medications.

    C. Incorrect: The family should be included when teaching about nonpharmacological treatments for agitation.

    D. **Correct:** Nonpharmacological treatments for agitation should always be used.

64. Answer is C (2B4)

    $15 \times 6 = 90$

    $90 \div 7.5 = 12$

    $12 \times 10 = 120$

    $120 \div 24 = 5$ mg/hour

65. Answer is B (4B5)

    A. Incorrect: These drugs do not belong to the hospice.

    B. **Correct:** The drugs should be disposed of by the hospice personnel (preferably the nurse who is responsible for medication management) and witnessed by a second individual as per the hospice's policy.

    C. Incorrect: These medications cannot be credited and therefore should not be returned to the pharmacy.

    D. Incorrect: These medications should be disposed of by the healthcare professional responsible for medication management.

66. Answer is C (4D3)

    A. Incorrect: Her behavior is normal for her age and not an indication of depression.

    B. Incorrect: Her behavior is normal and not a sign of disrespect for her mother's memory.

    C. **Correct:** Her behavior is normal for her age.

    D. Incorrect: Her grasp of concepts related to death, time, and permanence are limited and children her age often see death as temporary.

67. Answer is C (4D7)

    A. Incorrect: While the nurse can assist with notification that is not the purpose of the time of death visit.

    B. Incorrect: While the nurse can confirm the patient has died, the death certificate will require the signature of a physician or advanced practice registered nurse depending on state and/or local regulations.

    C. **Correct:** Comforting and supporting the family is a very important role of the hospice nurse at the time of death along with confirming the death and closure for the hospice staff member.

    D. Incorrect: This is not a purpose for attending the death of a hospice patient.

68. Answer is C (5C6)

    A. Incorrect: Clear communications are vital but the main role is to advocate for the patient's wishes.

    B. Incorrect: This is not the main role when communicating—this role would begin following the communication.

    C. **Correct:** This is the primary role of the nurse when communicating with the patient's physician.

    D. Incorrect: Suggestions are sometimes helpful but the main role of the nurse is patient advocacy.

69. Answer is D (6B4)

    A. Incorrect: This choice leaves out the family and patient and assumes coordination *for* rather than *with*.

    B. Incorrect: This choice leaves out the patient, family, and other health and human service providers.

    C. Incorrect: Decision-making is not the responsibility of one individual.

    D. **Correct:** Interdisciplinary collaborative practice includes all involved in the case including patient, family, other health or human service providers, and the interdisciplinary team (IDT).

70. Answer is A (7B2)

    A. **Correct:** This is the definition of beneficence.

    B. Incorrect: Veracity is truth telling.

    C. Incorrect: Nonmaleficence is avoiding the intentional infliction of harm.

    D. Incorrect: Justice is giving others what is due or owed and treating all people fair.

71. Answer is A (4B1)
    A. **Correct:** The core hospice team members providing services are nurses, physicians, medical social services, and counselors (spiritual or bereavement).
    B. Incorrect: The volunteer and hospice aide are not core members.
    C. Incorrect: The core team is specifically those listed in A. Other team members can be added as needed.
    D. Incorrect: The patient and family are not the core hospice team although they are certainly the focus of the core team's activity.

72. Answer is D (7A6)
    A. Incorrect: It would be inappropriate to contact the physician in this situation.
    B. Incorrect: Reacting in anger is unprofessional.
    C. Incorrect: The issue should be discussed and resolved by the parties involved—the nurse and the social worker. The supervisor should not be involved unless direct resolution efforts fail.
    D. **Correct:** Working directly with the social worker would be the best approach.

73. Answer is C (7A7)
    A. Incorrect: The Joint Commission does not require research.
    B. Incorrect: Research will help to find a cure for cancer but not all hospice and palliative care patients have a diagnosis of cancer.
    C. **Correct:** Research does improve the care of persons with serious and life-threatening illness. It is evidence-based outcomes that assure practice and treatment changes if recommendations have a scientific basis.
    D. Incorrect: Research is not responsible for making certain doctors will go along with the plan of care.

74. Answer is D (6B3)
    A. Incorrect: CD4 count must be less than 25 cells/mm^3.
    B. Incorrect: Advanced AIDS dementia complex is a supporting factor for hospice eligibility.
    C. Incorrect: Hospice eligibility criteria for human immunodeficiency virus (HIV) begin at 10%.
    D. **Correct:** A CD4 count of < 25 cells/mm^3 and a Karnofsky Performance score of ≤ 50% along with 1 of 9 additional criteria (of which a central nervous system [CNS] lymphoma is 1) meet hospice eligibility criteria for HIV.

75. Answer is D (3A6)
    A. Incorrect: Glucagon would be appropriate if the seizures were related to hypoglycemia.
    B. Incorrect: Antibiotics would be appropriate if the seizures were related to an infection.
    C. Incorrect: Supplemental oxygen would be appropriate if the seizures were related to hypoxemia.
    D. **Correct:** Additional fluids will decrease the effects of the high level of calcium.

76. Answer is A (2A3)

    A. **Correct:** Somatic pain is aching, constant, and well localized since it causes the activation of nociceptors in cutaneous and deep tissues.
    B. Incorrect: This is description of visceral pain.
    C. Incorrect: This is description of referred pain.
    D. Incorrect: This is a description of neuropathic pain.

77. Answer is B (2B5)

    A. Incorrect: Nonsteroidal anti-inflammatory drugs (NSAIDs) do inhibit platelet aggregation.
    B. **Correct:** NSAIDs are not antispasmodics.
    C. Incorrect: NSAIDs have analgesic benefits.
    D. Incorrect: NSAIDs do have antipyretic effects.

78. Answer is A (1B4)

    A. **Correct:** Dyspnea is the major symptom of type A COPD, emphysema. It is also a symptom of type B COPD, chronic bronchitis.
    B. Incorrect: Productive cough is a symptom of type B COPD.
    C. Incorrect: Central cyanosis is a symptom of type B COPD.
    D. Incorrect: Weight loss is seen with type A COPD.

79. Answer is D (2B4)

    $120 \times 2 = 240$

    $240 \times 0.1 = 24$ mg

80. Answer is D (3I3)

    A. Incorrect: Dehydration is truly considered a natural part of the dying process. To treat it would cause more discomfort due to ascites, nausea/vomiting, congestion, and the need to urinate more frequently.
    B. Incorrect: It cannot be arbitrarily stated that dehydration is never treated. Patient/family wishes are part of the decision process.
    C. Incorrect: Dehydration is not a medical emergency for a patient who is in the final phases of an illness.
    D. **Correct:** Dehydration is considered a part of the dying process. Not treating dehydration can decrease cough and congestion, edema and ascites, nausea and vomiting, and will decrease the frequency of urination, which can actually improve the quality of life. There may be times when hydration can relieve distressing symptoms (e.g., myoclonus).

81. Answer is A (1B6)

   A. **Correct:** Albumin levels decrease in end stage liver disease. Liver failure disables the function of protein catabolism.

   B. Incorrect: Encephalopathy is an early stage of hepatic coma.

   C. Incorrect: Coagulopathy is present due to the liver's inability to make clotting factors. This is especially dangerous when esophageal varices are present.

   D. Incorrect: Malnutrition is compounded by fatigue, alcohol intake, and ascites.

82. Answer is B (2B6)

   A. Incorrect: Addiction is a primary, chronic, neurobiologic disease, with genetic, psychosocial, and environmental factors influencing its development and manifestations.

   B. **Correct:** This is the correct definition of tolerance.

   C. Incorrect: Physical dependence is a state of adaptation that is manifested by a drug class-specific withdrawal syndrome that can be produced by abrupt cessation, rapid dose reduction, decreasing blood level of the drug, and/or administration of an antagonist.

   D. Incorrect: Pseudoaddiction is a result of undertreatment of pain causing the individual to appear to be a "drug seeker." In such cases, patients who have suffered prolonged, unrelieved pain may become more aggressive in seeking relief.

83. Answer is C (3D1)

   A. Incorrect: The patient's pattern of bowel movements should be maintained. Opioids decrease intestinal motility.

   B. Incorrect: If effective laxative agents are incorporated upon onset of opioid therapy, enemas should not be necessary.

   C. **Correct:** Opioids decrease intestinal motility therefore a bowel regimen should be initiated when opioid therapy begins.

   D. Incorrect: Although these efforts help with stool evacuation, they are insufficient with opioid administration.

84. Answer is A (3H8)

   A. **Correct:** Patients and families search for meaning of the individual's life and seek a purpose during the dying phase.

   B. Incorrect: Although financial concerns should never be minimized, the focus of the dying patient and their families is not the financial concerns.

   C. Incorrect: Hospice provides spiritual guidance to assist the patient and family in finding the meaning of life, but does not take care of "everything."

   D. Incorrect: Every care plan is individualized therefore no 2 are alike.

85. Answer is B (7A4)

   A.   Incorrect: Hospice offers symptom management; physical, emotional, psychosocial, spiritual, and bereavement care. Much is done to improve the quality of life for the individual and their family.

   B.   **Correct:** Hospice is a philosophy of care to improve quality of life for the terminally ill and their families.

   C.   Incorrect: Hospice is not a building although often there are inpatient hospice units/beds available for respite and/or acute symptom management.

   D.   Incorrect: Hospice is available 24 hours a day, 7 days a week.

86. Answer is B (6A4)

   A.   Incorrect: Palliative care can be delivered in any setting, but home is not the primary setting. Palliative care in the home in the final 6 months can be covered by the Medicare Hospice Benefit.

   B.   **Correct:** Palliative care is delivered primarily in the acute care settings either in a dedicated unit, outpatient clinic, or through palliative care teams.

   C.   Incorrect: Although nursing homes are perfect for the delivery of palliative care, the movement has far to grow in this setting.

   D.   Incorrect: Palliative care in the rehabilitation settings is rare, but would be appropriate in the circumstance of a patient who has a life-limiting progressively deteriorating disease.

87. Answer is D (4B2)

   A.   Incorrect: Most private insurance plans have a hospice benefit. For those that do not most will use a home health benefit or negotiate a rate for hospice.

   B.   Incorrect: See D.

   C.   Incorrect: See D.

   D.   **Correct:** If a program is Medicare certified, all patients must receive all the services available to a Medicare beneficiary whether or not the insurance company pays.

88. Answer is A (3J2)

   A.   **Correct:** Neutropenia is silent but dangerous leaving no neutrophils to fight the threat of infections. Neutropenia can be the cause of a septic situation, which is life-threatening.

   B.   Incorrect: Denudement of the gastrointestinal tract is usually very symptomatic with mouth ulcers, heartburn, nausea, and diarrhea.

   C.   Incorrect: Bone marrow suppression is a concern but it is the loss of neutrophils that creates the concern with the risk for overwhelming infections not anemia.

   D.   Incorrect: Anorexia and weight loss are very symptomatic causing great distress in the patient.

89. Answer is B (4B1)
    A. Incorrect: Palliative care does not have prognostic eligibility requirements.
    B. **Correct:** Although hospice requires a 6-month prognosis (should the disease run its usual course), palliative care does not.
    C. Incorrect: Eligibility for hospice care is directly related to prognosis.
    D. Incorrect: While functional status is part of prognosis, it is only 1 part of determining prognosis.

90. Answer is A (6B4)
    A. **Correct:** The patient and family are the unit of care for both hospice and palliative care.
    B. Incorrect: Care of the family is also part of both hospice and palliative care.
    C. Incorrect: Symptoms are not the unit of care—the patient and family is the unit of care.
    D. Incorrect: Reimbursement is not the focus of care in either hospice or palliative care.

91. Answer is C (4A1)
    A. Incorrect: When cure is possible, aggressive curative treatments are appropriate, if it is in keeping with the patient's goals of care.
    B. Incorrect: It is appropriate to suggest aggressive curative treatment when there is a realistic chance of worthwhile prolongation of life, if it is in keeping with the patient's goals of care.
    C. **Correct:** It is inappropriate to suggest aggressive curative treatment when the side effects of the treatment are more distressing than the potential benefits, if it is in keeping with the patient's goals of care.
    D. Incorrect: It is appropriate to suggest aggressive curative treatment when a patient chooses a clinical trial with informed consent, if it is in keeping with the patient's goals of care.

92. Answer is C (2B6)
    A. Incorrect: See C.
    B. Incorrect: They are not the same thing. Multifocal myoclonus can rarely occur with abstinence syndrome.
    C. **Correct:** Abstinence syndrome occurs when a person who is physically dependent on an opioid abruptly stops taking the opioid. It is a function of the elimination half-life of an opioid. The shorter the half-life, the sooner symptoms of abstinence syndrome will occur following the last dose of an opioid.
    D. Incorrect: Abstinence syndrome symptoms include anxiety, irritability, lacrimation, rhinorrhea, sweating, nausea, vomiting, diarrhea, abdominal cramps, insomnia, tachycardia, and elevated blood pressure.

93. Answer is C (3H10)

    A. Incorrect: This is a benefit of zolpidem, a non-benzodiazepine.
    B. Incorrect: This is a benefit of zolpidem, a non-benzodiazepine.
    C. **Correct:** Zolpidem does not treat anxiety. Lorazepam is a benzodiazepine.
    D. Incorrect: This is a benefit of zolpidem, a non-benzodiazepine.

94. Answer is B (2B2)

    A. Incorrect: See B.
    B. **Correct:** The baseline dose of long-acting opioids should be increased if more than 3 rescue doses are used in 24 hours.
    C. Incorrect: See B.
    D. Incorrect: See B.

95. Answer is B (3J3)

    A. Incorrect: Lymphedema can be a side effect of radiation therapy, especially in the treatment of breast cancer.
    B. **Correct:** Consult with physical or occupational therapists for their recommendation.
    C. Incorrect: Lymphedema is not related to cirrhosis.
    D. Incorrect: Using diuretics in patients with lymphedema may lead to volume depletion.

96. Answer is C (1BC)

    A. Incorrect: Colorectal cancer is the third leading cause of cancer death in men and women; 5-year survival of those with distant spread is less than 10%.
    B. Incorrect: Esophageal cancer is the sixth leading cause of death from cancer and occurs most frequently in those over the age of 50; overall 5-year survival rate in the United States is approximately 15%, with most people dying within the first year of diagnosis.
    C. **Correct:** The 5-year overall survival rate for hepatocellular cancer is 17% in the United States.
    D. Incorrect: Less than 24% of patients with pancreatic cancer survive longer than 1 year and 5-year survival is 5%; usually discovered in advanced stage; frequently resistant to chemotherapy and radiotherapy; fifth most common cause of cancer deaths in the United States.

97. Answer is A (2A1)

    A. **Correct:** Fears regarding addiction, tolerance, and diverse effects related to analgesics, particularly opioids, still persist.
    B. Incorrect: Instruction regarding pain during basic nursing education remains inadequate in most programs.
    C. Incorrect: Restrictive regulations, poor reimbursement, and lack of availability of treatments, especially opioids but also access to other therapies, markedly impede pain management.
    D. Incorrect: A pain scale alone does not give a complete pain assessment.

98. Answer is C (3B6)

    A. Incorrect: Tumor erosion from advanced head and neck cancer puts patients at high risk for hemorrhage.

    B. Incorrect: Hepatic failure causes decrease in clotting factors, and this can lead to hemorrhage.

    C. **Correct:** Patients are not at risk for hemorrhage even with advanced multiple myeloma.

    D. Incorrect: Low thrombocytes (platelets) can be an underlying cause of hemorrhage.

99. Answer is D (5A3)

    A. Incorrect: Determining how much his wife is involved in his mother's care is important, but not the initial response.

    B. Incorrect: Additional hospice aides may be needed, but further assessment of why he thinks he is doing a "horrible job" is needed.

    C. Incorrect: While it is good to validate his caregiving skills (if they are indeed great), telling him to move his mother to a nursing home is not appropriate.

    D. **Correct:** It is important to normalize his feelings and assess more about what he is feeling to help determine what can be done to help him.

100. Answer is B (2A2)

    A. Incorrect: This is the definition of hyperalgesia.

    B. **Correct:** This is the definition of allodynia.

    C. Incorrect: Painful muscle twitching involving the simultaneous contraction of contiguous groups of muscle fibers is the definition of muscle fasciculations.

    D. Incorrect: This is in part the definition of neuropathic pain.

101. Answer is A (3I1)

    A. **Correct:** Xerostomia is dry mouth and can be reversed or mitigated.

    B. Incorrect: Peritoneal carcinomatosis is a feature of the terminal phase of abdominal cancers.

    C. Incorrect: Increasing catabolism is a feature of end stage illness.

    D. Incorrect: Chemotherapy, while it may cause anorexia and weight loss, is not a cause of anorexia/cachexia syndrome (ACS) in end stage illness.

102. Answer is C (6A3)

   A. Incorrect: Continuous care is for a period of crisis when management of acute pain or other symptom is needed. When a caregiver who has been providing a skilled level of care for an individual becomes unable or unwilling to continue providing that care that may precipitate a crisis, however, continuous care would not be appropriate in situations where there are no acute pain management or other skilled needs.

   B. Incorrect: General inpatient care is provided in a hospital, skilled nursing facility, or hospice inpatient facility and is intended for the short-term management of pain or other symptoms that cannot reasonably be provided in the home setting.

   C. **Correct:** Respite care is inpatient care that is available to provide a needed rest for a caregiver who has become exhausted and/or unable to care for an individual at home. This level of care is provided in an inpatient setting for up to 5 calendar days.

   D. Incorrect: Most hospice care is routine home care. This is what the patient is receiving, but it does not provide 24-hour in-home care for the patient.

103. Answer is D (2B3)

   A. Incorrect: Rectal administration would cause more pain in a patient with anorectal pain.

   B. Incorrect: Patients with chronic leukemia often have thrombocytopenia and neutropenia.

   C. Incorrect: Patients with disseminated intravascular coagulation (DIC) may have widespread bleeding.

   D. **Correct:** The patient who is not able to take oral medication due to nausea and vomiting is appropriate for rectal medications.

104. Answer is C (3I4)

   A. Incorrect: This is a cause of fatigue.

   B. Incorrect: This is a cause of fatigue.

   C. **Correct:** Hypercalcemia can cause fatigue, not hypocalcemia.

   D. Incorrect: This is a cause of fatigue.

105. Answer is B (2B6)

   A. Incorrect: Gabapentin is an antiepileptic.

   B. **Correct:** Gabapentin is an adjuvant analgesic used to treat neuropathic pain.

   C. Incorrect: Pregabalin can provide an effect equivalent to gabapentin in lower doses.

   D. Incorrect: Gabapentin can be used by patients with renal failure.

106. Answer is A (2C3)

    A. **Correct:** Reiki is a Japanese technique that is administered by "laying on hands" and is based on the idea that an unseen "life force energy" flows through us and is what causes us to be alive.

    B. Incorrect: Similar to acupuncture, but instead of needles, pressure is used.

    C. Incorrect: Transcutaneous nerve stimulation uses low-voltage electrical current for pain relief.

    D. Incorrect: Massage is the manipulation of muscle and connective tissue.

107. Answer is D (3K2)

    A. Incorrect: Dementia develops more gradually and does not have a sudden onset.

    B. Incorrect: Nearing death awareness sometimes appears as confusion, but it usually is seen in persons nearing death.

    C. Incorrect: While possible, confusion would not be a likely indicator of progression of leukemia.

    D. **Correct:** A urinary tract infection (UTI) is likely. Older adults often do not present with a fever and sudden onset confusion is often a sign of infection in older adults.

108. Answer is B (4B4)

    A. Incorrect: With an average life expectancy of 41 years, homeless persons are 3 to 4 times more likely to die before those who are not homeless.

    B. **Correct:** Only 38% of homeless persons report having multiple chronic conditions.

    C. Incorrect: This is true as the patient goes back to being homeless.

    D. Incorrect: This is true.

109. Answer is C (2C1)

    A. Incorrect: This is inappropriate to say as it is contrary to what he just told you.

    B. Incorrect: Though difficult to accept, some people choose to be in pain in order to keep their cultural practices.

    C. **Correct:** This statement gives an opening to find what pain treatments are acceptable to him.

    D. Incorrect: This is not a correct statement.

110. Answer is C (3D2)

    A. Incorrect: While *Clostridium difficile* may cause diarrhea, it would not be the first step in assessment.

    B. Incorrect: Opioids commonly cause constipation not diarrhea.

    C. **Correct:** Use and overuse of dietary fiber, especially with decreasing food and fluid intake, often causes impaction, which could manifest itself as new onset diarrhea (liquid stool is able to pass the impaction).

    D. Incorrect: Complete bowel obstruction is characterized by constipation and an inability to pass flatus.

111. Answer is A (5A1)

   A. **Correct:** While this could be a case of emotional abuse, more information would need to be gathered before this is reported as a case of abuse.

   B. Incorrect: Any physical injuries not matching the stated cause needs to be investigated for abuse.

   C. Incorrect: It cannot be assumed that she is not reporting true events just because she has Alzheimer's disease. More assessment is needed immediately.

   D. Incorrect: This is a case of emotional abuse and action needs to be taken to ensure the patient's safety and adequate care.

112. Answer is C (2C3)

   A. Incorrect: Patients can be taught how to do self-hypnosis.

   B. Incorrect: Hypnosis has been proven to assist with pain management.

   C. **Correct:** Hypnosis is a mind–body therapy.

   D. Incorrect: This describes energy therapies like Reiki and healing touch.

113. Answer is D (3B4)

   A. Incorrect: Angina is experienced by over 0.5% of 20–39 year olds, 7.2% of 40–59 year olds, 14.7% of 60–79 year olds, and 21.1% of those 80 years of age and older.

   B. Incorrect: Definition of angina is chest pain or discomfort from inadequate blood flow to the heart muscle.

   C. Incorrect: Angina is a symptom of heart disease, which is the leading cause of death in the United States (nearly 598 000/year).

   D. **Correct:** Typical angina includes constricting discomfort in the anterior chest (e.g., tight, heavy, squeezing), neck, shoulders, jaw, and/or arms; it can be precipitated by physical exertion; and is usually relieved by rest or nitroglycerine in 5 minutes.

114. Answer is C (6B3)

   A. Incorrect: The first and second certification periods are for 90-day periods. Every subsequent certification period is 60 days. There is no limit on the number of times an individual may be recertified as long as they continue to meet eligibility criteria.

   B. Incorrect: Recertification does not change where a patient can receive hospice care.

   C. **Correct:** A hospice physician or hospice nurse practitioner (NP) must have a face-to-face encounter with each hospice patient prior to the beginning of the patient's third benefit period, and prior to each subsequent benefit period.

   D. Incorrect: Under the Medicare Hospice Benefit recertification, the same criteria are used for initial certification and recertification.

115. Answer is D (2B5)

   A. Incorrect: Not all types of pain can be treated with antidepressants.

   B. Incorrect: While all drugs need to be monitored for interactions, opioids can be used with antipsychotics.

   C. Incorrect: Uncontrolled symptoms such as intractable pain place patients at a greater risk for suicide.

   D. **Correct:** This is true.

116. Answer is D (3A7)

   A. Incorrect: Extrapyramidal symptoms (EPS) are not common with amyotropic lateral sclerosis (ALS).

   B. Incorrect: EPS is not common with chronic obstructive pulmonary disease (COPD).

   C. Incorrect: EPS is not common with multiple myeloma.

   D. **Correct:** EPS is common with Parkinson's disease.

117. Answer is A (1B9)

   A. **Correct:** Syndrome of inappropriate secretion of antidiuretic hormone (SIADH) results in abnormal laboratory values of a urine osmolality that is higher than plasma osmolality and elevated urinary sodium.

   B. Incorrect: SIADH is primarily associated with small cell lung cancer.

   C. Incorrect: SIADH is the inappropriate production of and secretion of the antidiuretic hormone causing *hypo*natremia.

   D. Incorrect: One of the treatments for SIADH is restricting free water to correct hyponatremia.

118. Answer is B (2A1)

   A. Incorrect: A furrowed brow *may* indicate pain.

   B. **Correct:** If the pain behaviors stop or lessen after the trial of an analgesic, then the presence of pain has been confirmed.

   C. Incorrect: Vocalizations *may* indicate pain.

   D. Incorrect: Unconscious patients do feel pain.

119. Answer is B (3A6)

   A. Incorrect: Phenothiazines lower the seizure threshold.

   B. **Correct:** Haloperidol does not lower the seizure threshold.

   C. Incorrect: Tricyclic antidepressants lower the seizure threshold.

   D. Incorrect: Tramadol lowers the seizure threshold.

120. Answer is A (5B2)

   A. **Correct:** The patient has been living with not being able to read for a long time and would have ways to work around it.

   B. Incorrect: This may not be practical and would leave the patient still not knowing her medication regimen.

   C. Incorrect: This could be seen as punitive to the patient; rote memory does not equate to understanding.

   D. Incorrect: She would still need to understand the times and this would only work until her medications are changed.

121. Answer is D (1B1)

   A. Incorrect: Bony lytic lesions are seen in multiple myeloma and are rare in lymphoma.

   B. Incorrect: Lynch syndrome is seen in solid tumor cancers.

   C. Incorrect: *BRCA2* gene is a mutation that is a risk factor for breast cancer.

   D. **Correct:** Lymphomas (Hodgkin's and non-Hodgkin's) with a T-cell origin are known to be most aggressive in progression.

122. Answer is B (3I5)

   A. Incorrect: See B.

   B. **Correct:** Fatigue is the most common symptom, followed by pain, terminal secretions/noisy breathing, delirium, dyspnea/cough, and urinary incontinence/retention.

   C. Incorrect: See B.

   D. Incorrect: See B.

123. Answer is D (5A3)

   A. Incorrect: Caution should be used when viewing any teaching materials on websites that are interested in selling products. See D.

   B. Incorrect: See D.

   C. Incorrect: See D.

   D. **Correct:** No matter the source, nurses should only recommend teaching materials from websites that they have viewed themselves.

124. Answer is B (6B6)

   A. Incorrect: See B.

   B. **Correct:** Volunteer service hours must account for 5% of all direct patient care hours for all paid hospice employees and contract staff in a Medicare certified hospice program.

   C. Incorrect: See B.

   D. Incorrect: See B.

125. Answer is D (3C4)

   A. Incorrect: With aspiration pneumonia, percussion is likely normal with audible crackles.

   B. Incorrect: Chronic bronchitis produces resonant sounds on percussion.

   C. Incorrect: Metastatic lesions are rarely large enough to cause widespread dullness on percussion.

   D. **Correct:** With pleural effusion, the exam will likely reveal decreased breath sounds on auscultation on the affected side, reduced transmission of the voice to the chest wall (vocal fremitus), and stony dullness on percussion.

126. Answer is D (1B3)

   A. Incorrect: Confronting a patient with the "truth" is rarely appropriate. What appears as "denial" is often something else including a lack of information or understanding.

   B. Incorrect: American College of Cardiology/American Heart Association (ACC/AHA) stage D indicates advanced disease.

   C. Incorrect: While this may be a possibility, the patient's prognosis would make it unlikely he would be able to travel a year from now.

   D. **Correct:** What appears as "denial" is often something else, including a lack of information or understanding.